POTTY TRAINING FOR BOYS AND GIRLS IN THREE DAYS

The Step-by-Step Plan

ANNA ANNISTON

TABLE OF CONTENTS

POTTY BOYS TRAINING

As far as potty training is concerned, there is a gender disparity between boys and girls. Although some fundamentals remain the same, there are typically significant variations between potty boys and girls. Know the secrets of potty training and appreciate these nuances to make your child a potty training professional with less tension and disappointment.

When you start potty training, it depends on the specific child. However, before you start toilet training, there are several things to remember.

Many girls may be prepared for potty training as young as 18 months old, or may not be fully prepared for potty training until they are four.

Children seem to be ready for potty training when it comes to taking their time. They're usually a couple of months behind girls, and many aren't ready until they're two years old at first.

Keep in mind that every child is unique. Your older son will be a potty superstar, starting 18 months of toilet training. Your daughter may not be able to start until she's two, and your younger son won't react until he's three. Potty boy training can be a hard job, especially as the males appear to be the stubbornest of both sexes. I just didn't make it up; it's real! Studies show that girls sometimes take a few weeks to complete potty training faster than boys. Nonetheless, I have some ideas that will help you train your boy even faster than other children. This is also a case of knowing children's psychology and seeking to cultivate a desire for a potty education in the children's eyes. It sounds complicated, but it's straightforward.

This is a good tip for teaching him potty

You need to produce a want to teach the child potty. This means talking and communicating and trying to develop his interests at his level. The most straightforward approach is to deal with something he loves, trusts, or likes to watch on TV! Am I thinking here about toys-has he got a favorite teddy bear? If so, this is your arsenal's hidden weapon to help your kid potter faster.

Use the tool to speak to him at a point he understands. Give your visual demonstrations and the pet, and in no time will you have him educated potty. **It doesn't have to take Long Potty Training!**

Is one month the average time a boy takes to be fully trained-do you have more than a month to train your kid potty, or would you prefer to travel faster? There is no good reason why you can't be fully trained in a few days if you can genuinely understand child psychology. The last thing I can suggest is to enjoy the moment and make sure that you treat it as an accomplishment when your boy gets completely potted.

How to demonstrate the proper powerful technique

Some children learn better when they see what they can do in the bowl. Kids should watch Mama, but Daddy is not generally interested in this potty-watching phase in his daughter's training.

Dad really should get interested now. Kids will watch father go potty. Even if you begin by teaching your son to do his whole business while he's sitting, Dad can still demonstrate. Boys will react to the feeling that they want to be like Daddy and see how things work.

New Parents Quick Potty Training

Make sure your child does not get constipated. This is the most critical start. Children fear the toilet and into a cold, wet small room. If you are not an expert on constipation, call the doctor if you see signs that you don't eat well or that you change the mood. Increase your regular intake of fluids and vitamins. Water plays a vital role in making it easier for your child to remain healthy and digest. Give plenty of water and allow them to drink with encouragement. Children can enrich fiber: Barley, Navy Bohemian, Baked Beans, Split Peas, Oat Bran, Raspberries, Green Peas, Purple, Broccoli, Mixed Vegetables, Strawberries, Carrots, Potatoes, Corn, Rice, Apples, Oranges, Celery.

Learn your child's potty training storybooks. Many books are available online for potty training. Reading and imagining help the child respond to and observe the fascinating features and actions of the story. Provide plenty of attention if your child succeeds. It's not an easy task, but it will allow you to see great results when you truly make your child proud.

Avoid physical punishment if the potty is not used. Replace the memories with your child's potty training stories. It helps them to understand the story and how they understand it when it's time.

Throw away clothes and pull-ups and go on as soon as possible. Perform so as soon as possible, because this will speed up the whole operation. Help them to avoid easing themselves, relying on the diapers. A change of clothing will make them feel bigger. Support your child with their potty chair secure. Only let your kid spend time with the potty. Give them toys while sitting on the pot and the diapers on so that they can easily play with them before using them. Bound foods such as rice, bananas, corn, cheese, and citrus juice to constipate. Take your child first in the morning to the potty and thirty minutes after a complete meal. Read books, tell a story, sing a song or talk, it will help you relax. Tell your child to take a few deep breaths and get them to close their eyes while talking or singing. Enjoy soothing music while sitting potty. And don't worry if they're not doing well, because it takes time for anything.

How to show a proper potty technique

Most children learn faster when they see what they can do in the potty.

Dad really should get interested now. Children will watch Dad go potty. Even if you begin by teaching your son to do all while sitting, Dad can still demonstrate. Boys will react to the feeling that they want to be like Papa and see how things work.

The potty training cycle separates boys and girls once more when it comes to discipline and interest. The most important thing you need to consider is to preserve your composure regardless so that your children will not be overwhelmed by feelings that turn potty training into a traumatic experience. Most boys think that they have better things to do than go potty, and their endurance is faster, and their interest in potty training is faster. Initially, they can also be enthusiastic about potty training and lose interest the same day.

Watching the signs of a frustrated potty trainer, modifying the methods, or even postponing potty training is crucial.

PRE POTTY TRAINING: THE POTTY TRAINING STEPS

Before beginning your child's potty training, you would expect numerous outlets to provide information and tips on this process. Parenting newspapers, family, friends and experts are some of the outlets. Many approaches and a variety of advice are available to facilitate this mission. The primary requirement is to choose a program that is suitable for you and your kids. If you have two children, you don't need to use one technique for both. You might have to use one program for one child and a completely different program for another child.

Some parents typically don't want to train their children until they reach two years of age. You wait until your child speaks the words synonymous with toiletries.

On the other hand, some kids can train at this age quickly, and some create issues because they want to do whatever they want when a child turns two.

When you say, "It's time to go potty," they generally refuse because they didn't want this thing to do like this. Another thing that will worry about the child's trainer before he fulfills his wish.

As the child grows up, it becomes challenging to convince them to stay on the potty for an extended period. A child can begin to play instead of taking the time to stop and use the potty.

One of the significant drawbacks of late potty training is that children who are entirely prepared for potty typically require pre-schools. This delay prevents the infant from being enrolled in the children's school on time, which is essentially a detriment for the entirety of his educational career.

Families should recognize their child's signs associated with toilet activities such that they are the only ones who can contribute a significant amount to potting training. Parents should also be careful not to prolong their child's potty training.

Many of us try refreshment during the hot days, but this pee trick is not one of them when your kid sits on your shoulders. At one point or another, we all fall victim to catching our children as their clothes raising the white flag and unveiling the contents on our lap. But we get into potting training with fists clenched and Clint Eastwood-like resolve. However, this isn't just a walk in the park either.

They have to learn to crawl and then walk before they learn to run. The same pattern of growth applies to potty training. What many dads don't know, though, is that there are many drills and activities for their kids in the months leading up to potty training that will ease the process when the time comes.

Such activities will also introduce you to the new engine and cognitive skills, which will lead to your overall growth.

There are many reasons why potty training is a problem for young children. First of all, the act of going to the toilet requires several different steps.

Children must go from an easy and reasonable step to understand the urge to the run-up to the potty undressing to sit down, and then, then, and only then, will they do what they'd do mercilessly before: pee.

All these steps have to be taken in their precise order to confuse the matter further. For example, if a young child were to sit down and then attempt to take his or her pants off, it would possibly never get past his or her underwear. While this is what you may have done on a drunken night, we can assure you it will be much less' fresh.'

Finally, children succeed if they take all the steps correctly. They miss the target if they skip one of them or plan to alter one. Consider that your little one wanted to go to the next potted plant, but they did all the rest correctly. Your philodendron may like the fertilizer, but we think you will not enjoy cleanup.

Pre Potty Training Steps

The children should be taught lessons before dumping the diaper, to solve the difficulties of the multi-step phase of potty training.

1. Learning how to get rid of The first lesson is how to get rid of it. Undressing is better than dressing and is an ideal starting point. This requires the same motor skills, which delivers results more rapidly. Moreover, if the impulse hits, the fewer barriers they have to tackle, the more often they succeed.

   When it's time to become pajamas or go into the bathroom, begin to teach them to undress. The first step is to learn how to move pants or lift a dress: feel free to weave your dressing skills, and do not be afraid to become involved!

   Show them the difference between their pants ' front and back.

   Let them put your socks on your feet and change your socks to do the same. Tell them how to wear regularly, to include them in the dressing process, so that they have some influence over their wardrobe.

   Perhaps you could even compete with your child to see who can dress up first!

2. Another very critical part of this puzzle is to expose your child to multi- step directions. World of Moms claims that when your child is turned into an infant, "Between 18 and 24

months, a baby will learn as many as 50 new words a week. When his thinking starts to change, his mind continues to keep track of daily events. That's the prime age for giving children2-stage directions. "pre potty training, daddy, modern paternity, potty training. The two or three-stage guidance should assist the children in managing procedures rather than individual activities. Good times are during exercise, meals, or clean-up to do this workout. You can tell your boy, for example: to pick up his truck and then do a puzzle with him.

Sit down and wash her hands for lunch.

Only put his shoes at the front door, and you're going to play cards.

When learning the ability to follow multiple steps, "use the potty, then we go for a walk," this is a reasonable requirement, not an overwhelming one.

3. Pre-potty exercise–think about it!

Finally, think about the bathroom in the months before you plan potty training. Consider it part of your daily talks. It helps make anything in the bathroom open and relaxed and not fabulous. Allow your child to enter the bathroom with you to make the toilet a regular part of your day. As Parents, we love the temple that is the toilet bathroom, and throne. Feed your little one with passion!

You should clarify that when they are a little bigger, they will begin to piss and fuck into the toilet. Choose ordinary pee and poop phrases. How these words do not matter, but it is essential to use similar words and use them consistently. When these terms become more relevant, it helps to reduce confusion.

By exposing them to reading and other toilet games, you teach them that patience is an essential component for success.

Please find out after you have finished washing your hands to get rid of germs. And what do you know?

Congratulations, and celebrate your achievements. For a moment, you've done a great deal with one of your poops. Create a walk of victory and take your little one on the journey.

They have to learn to crawl and then walk before they learn to run. The same pattern of growth applies to potty training. Before they learn to master the potty, they must first learn the pretty potty skills to use porcelain. Well done, Papa. Well done. Your little one's going to be in the potty early enough. And the rest of life, as we all know, is downhill.

THE THREE-DAY POTTY TRAINING TECHNIQUE

For children under three who are ready for potty trains and for parents who can spend a long weekend on potty training, this strategy will save their lives. Julie Fellom, the preschool instructor, has developed the very successful Diapers Free Toddler program, but you can try other similar approaches.

The idea that a few days or even one afternoon from your child could be comfortable with the potty sounds too good to be true, isn't it?

Although this can sound crazy if one expects long and complicated potty training, "quick training" works for many parents. Here we explain the "three-day potty training" technique in the Diaper Free Toddlers program of

Julie Fellom and send you step-by-step guidance on how it works for you. One thing to bear in mind: even though your child uses the pot instead of diapers, he may still encounter accidents.

After practicing potty, more than 200 children began Diaper Free Toddlers, an instructor of pre-school in San Francisco, in 2006. The primary purpose was to remove discarded clothes from savings by encouraging parents to educate their children earlier. Fellom says her approach will work for children as young as 15 months of age, and for those younger than 28 months, it is most effective.

Fellom says that children may be more prone to potty training after this period. "Working for children who try it before 28 months is guaranteed," says Fellom. "The closer you hit the age of 3, the less likely it is to succeed." After a potty training weekend at home, children can go to the potty for punching or pooping consistently and have few incidents, says Fellom.

Are you set for potty workouts?

The technique of Fellom includes attention, concentration, and dedication. This is a "bar-bottomed" approach that ensures your child will have to be bare under her tail for three months after starting a potty workout and wear loose-fitting pants with nothing below her while she's out or in daycare.

It is all right to use diapers and training pants for bedding and snacks, but if you depend on them too often, you can reverse the success of your potty training, says Fellom.

What you need for your potty exercise weekend Treats that encourage peeing–oily, soak or foods with high water content such as watermelon and popsicles (in addition to daily nutritious meals) Supply chairs that you use at home–values for any principal place where you spend time, plus any toilet. According to Fellom, this includes: to remain dry for at least two hours at a time.

Demanding your potty to wear slides

Each day to periodically clear your schedule and intend for a whole weekend based on potty training. This ensures that you cancel all your daily weekend events and make sure that your potty training partner is still around for at least the first two days to help.

Give your potty training buddy a "potty dance." The purpose is to celebrate the achievements of your child and to encourage it to continue, so the dance can range from a tweaked end-zone chicken dance to a complete rumba with accompanying music–anything that feels good to you.

Begin to teach your child about the potty. Two to five weeks before your weekend's potting training, each time you, your wife, or another family member needs to go to the bathroom and take your children along to observe the process, including how to remove their pants and underwear. Sit on the potty Pee or fall into it.

Purchase several potty chairs or rent some. Put a potty in your home in every main room and bathroom.

Have your child ready to dip the diapers. The week before you begin, show your kid a pile of slides and explain that she will soon no longer need to wear them, because she can go home naked for a while. Present it as an exciting and enjoyable development (if your child is at least two).

How to teach potty in three days:

DAY1: Get up with your kid when he wakes up. For the remainder of the day, make him go under the waist naked.

Take turns to watch your child with your potty training partner for signals that he wants to pink or punch. When he starts to go, carry him to the potty quickly as you say, "Pee goes to the potty." Salt and watery treats, drink plenty of water, so everyone should sometimes pink, throughout the day.

Celebrate the progress of your child when the quantity of pee (even a few drops) or poop hits the potty instead of the floor. Do the potty dance when this happens. You may also pay tribute, high-five, etc.

When your child has a spill, say, "Pee (or poop) goes to the potty," as you are purifying it. Never scream at him or taunt him because accidents are going to happen.

Tell your child it's time to go potty before bed and snack. (Don't ask your child because he probably says no.) Put a slide on your child before he sleeps, if you feel confident he'll stay dry.

Day 2: Follow the day one direction.

During nap time in day 2, when your child has peeled in the potty, take a short walk outside altogether. Plan to quit no more than 30 minutes, and carry you a potty.

Have your child wear loose pants, without any socks or bras.

Day three: follow the guidelines for day one. (Take your child's extra clothes when you are not fortunate enough to get them accident-free home.) During nap time, leave for roughly 30 minutes (as on day two).

Just before you leave the house, let your child use the potty every time. Wear your child in loose pants without anything below.

Carry a change of clothes and a small travel pot if your child wants to go out. After your kid's potty training weekend, you might expect your child to start getting a little pee in the potty 10-12 times when they have to go. But to step up the contract, some follow-up has to be done: while you are home for the next three months, make your child go naked below the waist. (You should dress your child in loose pants with nothing underneath while she is not at home–even at daycare).

Let your child start wearing lightweight, loose-fitting underwear after three months without incident. At this point, she doesn't have to go homeless!

Hold a portable travel potty in the car and note the public bathroom nearest you to and fro.

And if you don't have the hang of using the potty after your potty exercise weekend, simply wait one month or two, then try again

The upside of potty training in three days

A potty training weekend can be convenient and easy to follow the way to start the cycle (or wait until your child is two if she is younger than this). If you were scared of potty education, stressed about how to proceed, or wondered how to teach your child to use potty instead of just sitting on it, this solution could be a holy end.

Contrary to other methods, the process works quickly, even with follow-up and retrogress.

You will save time and frustration for yourself. Your child is proud of his success and freedom.

By removing diapers sooner, you can save money and protect the environment.

You will not have to give your child the money to use the potty because there are no therapies or other incentives (other than a potty dance).

Powerful training and excitation will benefit a kid who has avoided the potty or never showed interest by dancing exuberantly any time a little pee or poop transforms it into the potty.

The downside to potty training in three days is usually three days at home, as you watch the step of your child and whisk it to the potty. It can be daunting for two working parents to commit themselves to potty training on the same day.

It can be a struggle to complete the follow-up process, depending on your childcare situation. Providers may not be willing or able to keep your child out of the slides, underwear, and pants during treatment.

If you're interested in accelerated potty training, here are some other ideas that might make the process work best for you: use other incentives, like sticks, therapies, or promises of big kid's underwear, rather than a potty dance.

Use a doll to demonstrate peeing at the toilet, instead of taking your child to your bathroom. Less Than a Day's Toilet Learning demonstrates how to do this.

THE POTTY TRAINING ABCs.

Many parents welcome toilet exercises as a landmark in the growth of their children–though it means nothing but an end to growing pains. But few mothers and dads are ready for the duration of toilet training.

Some children will master it in a couple of days, while some will take several months or longer. When you understand the essential elements of training before you begin, you and your child are better prepared to succeed. Below are the necessary steps:

A. **Assess** the readiness of your child–and your own

B. **Buy** the right equipment.

C. **Create** a routine.

D. **Demonstrate** to your child

E. **Explain** the process

F. **Frequently** Encourage habit

G. **Grab** any pants of preparation

H. **Handle setbacks gracefully**

I. **Introduce** preparation at night

J. **Jump for joy!** You're done!

A. Evaluate the readiness of your child–and your own Once children are about one year old; they will begin to see that the rectum or bladder is full. Many people can start potty training as early as 18 months, while others are still involved after three years. Many parents start potty training when their children are approximately 2 1/2.

As the age spectrum of children who are involved in potty training is so broad, look for signs that your kid is ready to begin: can she obey basic instructions? Could she sit and walk? Will she take her pants off and put them on again? Try not to push her–it's just counterproductive if she's not ready.

And don't expect your child to have the same schedule as your older child. Children tend to train a bit slower than boys, whereas the second (and subsequent) learn faster than the firstborn.

Consider the other challenges now faced by your kid. If she is in trouble or has big changes in her life, such as a new school, nurse, or parent, the cycle of potty training would possibly hit some snags. Try waiting before things get resolved.

The same goes for you: if you've just taken a tough new job in your house, or have morning sickness with the next pregnancy, it's probably not a good time to try to train your child. Wait a few weeks–or months–to ease other stresses. Prepare a potty training if you or the primary carers of your child will spend time, patience, and fun in the process. And be prepared for several months for potty training.

B. First of all, invest in a children's potty chair or a special adapter seat that suits your standard toilet. This will make kids feel less nervous about using the adult toilet–some of them fear falling into it while others don't like the sudden flush noise.

Find out what equipment your child needs before you go shopping and then ask him to help you pick a potty chair. Write down his name and invite him to play with it when you get home.

When you buy a potty chair for your baby, look for one with or without a ward with a removable urine shield. You may need to clean up a little more spilled pee, but when he sits on the bowl, the guards appear to scratch the penis of a young boy and prevent him from practicing.

If you use the adapter bench, make sure it is comfortable and stable and buy a stool to go with it. The kid wants a stool to get up and down quickly and conveniently from the toilet and to grip the feet when sitting.

C. Place the child in a potty, fully dressed position once a day–before bed, bath, or if she has a bowel movement. Create a routine. It helps her to get used to the potty and embrace it. If there isn't a bathroom nearby, carry your child's portable potty outside or to your playroom or wherever she usually's. After that routine is all right, make her sit on the bare-bottomed potty. Finally, let her get used to what it feels like. Now, please let her know it is grown-up to remove your pants before wearing the bowl because this is what Mommy and Daddy (and any older siblings) do every day.

If you sit on the potty with or without your child's shoes, don't force it. Never stop her or force her physically to sit down, mainly if she seems afraid. It is safer for a couple of weeks to set the pot aside before trying again. So, if she is happy to sit there, you know that she's relaxed enough to go ahead.

D. Prove for your child that children learn by imitation, and watching you use the bathroom is a standard way of learning everything about the use of the toilet. If you have a son, teaching him to sit at first is more comfortable. He can watch his father, older brother, or friend stand up when he has mastered it–he is bound to hang it quickly with just some encouragement.

When you show your child how you know the time to go to the bathroom is helpful. So explain what happens when you use the bathroom and then let it look in the bathroom. Furthermore, show him how you wipe your underwear, flush your toilet, and wash your hands.

Even though you'll support your child for some time with these activities, particularly wiping after a bowel motion, watching you do it and hearing it talk allows him to get familiar with the entire process. (If your child is a female, help her wipe from the front and back to reduce the risk of urinary tract infections, especially after a bowel movement.) If your child has older siblings or friends with high-quality schooling, consider showing them as well. This can be good for your child to see someone close to your age, demonstrating his or her skills.

E. Explain the process. Show your child the link between toilet and pooping. If she poops into her drawing the next time, carry her up to the potty, sit down and dump the pain into the tub. Have her flush, if she wishes, and she can watch her feces disappear. You may also want to pick up some picture books or videos on potty training. (Don't push her if she is afraid.) Taro Gomi's

Everybody Poops is a longtime favorite, and even Where is the Poop? And once on a Potty, also a doll and miniature potty version. Keeping such a book in a bathroom or a poster or flipbook showing the steps to using the potty will help your child remember all of this new knowledge and familiarize him/her with the procedure.

F. Encourage your child to sit on the pot when he feels the urge to go. If he wants support to get there and take off his slide, make sure that he knows that it's all right to ask you anytime.

When you can, occasionally let him run around bare-bottomed with the nearby potty. The more time he spends on diapers, the faster he can know (although you will need to wipe up some more puddles). Tell him he can use the potty anytime he wants, and occasionally ask him if he needs it.

Often children won't sit on the potty long enough to relax. Encourage your child gently to live for at least one or two minutes. If you keep him company and talk to him or read him a book, you could be better off.

If your child successfully uses the potty, showed him love and give him positive reinforcement as he practices potty training. Sometimes he will start with mistakes, but he will begin to realize that bringing something into the pot is an achievement.

(Just try not to do anything on any potty ride, or your child will be anxious and self-confident.)

G. Grab some pants After exercise, consider adding pants to your routine. Training pants, which pull on and off like underwear, are disposable or cloth diapers. They allow your child to unwrap the potty alone, which is a critical step towards being fully potted.

Although cloth training pants are less comfortable than pull-ups on the floor, many parents believe they work better because your child can feel when she pees or pulls. Whatever choice you choose, slowly –perhaps just a couple of hours at a time –add them and stick with slides at night.

When your child consistently looks for the potty whenever she has to go, it's time to move on to "big-kid" underwear. Many moms and dads have found that undies with a favorite character on them encourage kids to stay dry.

H. **Handle setbacks gracefully:** Toilet training can be difficult for parents and children. Keep in mind that temporary setbacks are entirely normal, and virtually every child will have several accidents before being able to stay dry all day long. An accident doesn't mean that you've failed. When it happens, don't get angry or punish your child. After all, it's only recently that his muscle development has allowed him to hold his bladder and rectum closed at all, and he's still learning why it's essential to use the potty. Mastering the process will take time.

What can you do? Reduce the chance of accidents by dressing your child in clothes that are easy to remove quickly. When he has an accident anyway, be positive and loving and calmly clean it up. Suggest sweetly that next time he try using his potty instead.

I. **Introduce night training**: Don't offer the stash of diapers yet. Even when your child is clean and dry all day long, it may take a few more months, or even years, to keep her dry all night long. At this age, her body is still too untimely to reliably wake her to the bathroom in the middle of the night. It is common for children to wet the bed thoroughly into grade school.

Keep your child in a painting or pull-up at bedtime before beginning a night training course, but allow her to use the potty if she needs pee or shower at night. Tell her that she can call you for help if she wakes up in the middle of the night. You can also try to put her pot close to her bed so that she can use it right there.

If she seems to stay dry always at night, night training could be an excellent time to start. To cover the mattress, place a plastic sheet under the fabric. Put the kid in underwear (or nothing) and use the toilet before tucking it in. See how it goes, then. When she wakes up, get her to use the toilet before her day begins.

Mind that many children can't stay dry until their school-age at night. Bed- wetting is unintentional, and children have no control. If you can't get dry overnight, put her back in the night diapers to make sure that she doesn't get to bed weather and try again when she's a little older in a few months.

J. Jump for joy, you are done! Believe it or not, whether your child can master this new ability emotionally and physically, it does. And if you wait for it to start, it shouldn't be too difficult for anyone of you.

Once it is over, affirm your pride in the accomplishment by encouraging him to support a family of younger kids with remaining diapers or help you pack clothes and send them away for the last time with a cloth delivery service.

And don't forget to pat on the back. You will never have to worry about diapers again, anyway, for this guy!

The best time to start potty training your son. Your son's teaching how to use the potty needs him to help and inspire, along with time and patience.

Five potty training strategies

Let him watch and learn to imitate the girls, and it is a reasonable first step to watch you use your bathroom. He can note that Daddy uses the potty differently from mummy so that you can illustrate the simple mechanics of how boys use the toilet.

Be anatomically accurate when speaking of body parts. If you do not use a dumb name to call his penis a pee-pee for some other body section, it may mean that the genitals are disgusting.

When your child sits on the potty, he needs to be able to lean on the ground with his feet, particularly when his bowel is moving slightly. Most experts suggest the purchase of a children's pot that your child can say for themselves, and that will also feel better than sitting in a full-size toilet. (Many kids fear falling into the toilet, and their anxiety can interfere with potty training.) Make sure it is comfortable and firmly installed if you want to purchase an adapter seat for your regular toilet. Get a shack for your son, too, so that he can quickly get on and off the potty any time with his feet.

When you purchase a potty for your baby, check for one without a urine guard (or a removable one). Although they will shield your bathroom from a tiny stray pee, they also appear to scratch the penis when a boy sits on the toilet, which may make him reluctant to use it.

You may want to display pictorial books or videos relevant to your son to try to help him appreciate all these new details. All Poops is a favorite forever, by Taro Gomi, just like Uh, Yeah! Have to Go! Have to Go! By Bob McGrath and Alona Frankel Once Upon a Potty, which comes with a doll and a miniature potty.

Help your child become confident with the potty. Let your children get used to the concept of the potty. Begin by telling him the potty is his own. You may customize it by writing your name or allowing it to be decorated with stickers. Then try to lie with his clothes on it.

After a week or so in this way, suggest that he try it out with his pants. If it seems resistant at all, stop the temptation to move it. It can only lead to a power struggle that could ruin the entire process.

Use this for potty demonstrations if your child has a favorite doll or stuffed animal. Many kids like to watch their toy move about, so your child will learn more than what to do by showing him.

Some parents also build a doll or stuffed animal toilet. Your child can be hanging on his potty, but his toy can sit on its own.

Motivate him with fresh underwear Educate your son on the advantages of being raised by sending him on a particular order to buy big boy underwear. Let him know that he has the alternative (animals or trains, briefs, or boxers, whatever appeals he wants).

Plan the outing so that he is excited to be old enough to wear the "actual" underwear like the potty one of his dad or older brother. When he appears reluctant to put them on, see if he's going to wear them on his slide. Once he becomes accustomed to them, he may insist on the disposable.

Establish a training plan To exclude your child from slides depends on your daily routine and whether your son is in daycare or pre-school. If he is, you may want to communicate with his daycare provider or professor about your plan.

You'll have to decide whether to turn to underwear full time or change between diapers and underwear. Disposable training pants are comfortable, but many experts and parents find it safer to change to underwear or old-fashioned cotton pants, allowing your son instantly to feel when wet. For example, that ensures that some events will be washed.

Remember what's best for you and your son when making your decision. Your doctor may recommend one or the other form. Continue to use diapers or disposable pants for a while at night and while you are out. The childcare provider or pre-school teacher may have her ideas on when to turn to school babies.

Teach him to sit down first, then bowel movements and urine always come concurrently, so it makes sense to have your son sit down to pee. He discovers that both go to the potty in this way. He will not also be distracted by the fun of spraying and learning when you need him to focus on mastering the necessary procedure.

Don't let him stay too long (15 minutes is enough) or be distracted by other things. Watching TV or other screens while sitting on the potty is often a big obstacle for parents and children.

When your son is relaxed sitting down to the toilet, he will try to stand up. (There's no need to hurry–he can continue to pee as long as he likes.) Getting a male role model is essential here.

Make sure your son can take his father, his uncle, or a good family friend into the bathroom to see him stand up. If your son seems to have the idea, let him try it.

If he seems unwilling, try to put some O-shaped cereal into the potty for target practice. Expect a few masses to clean up while your son is perfecting his mission. When you don't hesitate to let him pee in the yard, you can paint a mark on a tree or code the mark.

Take naked time away. Nothing helps your baby to find out if he needs to go for a while in the nude. Place the potty in an accessible area when he plays and allow him to sit there frequently.

(Whether your child is playing naked, be prepared for the floor to muddy. Let your child play in a damp space or put plastic on the tapes and furniture.) Look for signs that he must go, like catching himself or jumping on and off, and use these signals to indicate that it might be a potty time. You can do it on a few days in a row, in the evenings while your family is together, or on weekends. The longer your child spends on slides, the more he learns.

Celebrate victories. Your son may have a few mistakes, but he will finally be able to get everything in the pot. Celebrate with fanfare this moment.

Reinforce the belief that he accomplished an essential achievement, for example, by rewarding him with a "big child," like watching a new video or staying on the playground for longer.

Remember not to do a lot on every trip to the potty. Otherwise, your child will feel stressed and aware of everything.

If it's not effective at first, try again. As in all other things, the more the potty he uses, the easier it is. Yet you should do other things to make it easier for him.

Put your child in loose clothing, which he can take away easily, or buy underwear of too big a size.

Don't overreact or threaten if he still has problems with potty training. Nothing can interfere with potty training quicker than making a child feel guilty after an accident.

If you feel irritated, remind yourself that it could mean months to wet your child's pants. Recall that potty training is less than learning to ride a bike, and accidents are an inevitable part of the process. Even kids who have regularly used the bathroom for months sometimes have an incident when they are involved.

And it's perfectly reasonable to stop from training potty and try again in a couple of weeks if you don't feel much progress or if you or your kid is frustrated.

Increase the fun factor Your child would be more inspired if you treat potty training with a little pizzazz.

Drip some coloring blue food into the potty. Your child will be amazed by how he can green the water. In the magazine rack next to the toilet, place some of his favorite books so he can look at them whenever he wants to go. And even better, read (if not a distraction) to him. Perhaps he would like to cut shapes out of toilet paper for target practice.

You may want to consider providing incentives if your child continues to lose interest but is well into potty training.

One common approach is to use stickers and a calendar to keep track of his achievements. He gets a sticker every time he goes to the potty that he can fit on the page. Watching the stickers stack up will inspire him.

When there is no anticipation for the stickers, you can give a more incentive such as a delicacy from the candy aisle in the supermarket or a toy if it gets enough stickers or remains dry for several days in a row.

Going into night mode, You should start formulating a game plan for the night when your son is dry all day long. Wait until he uses the potty reliably during the day, and check his slides in the mornings and after the naps for dryness. In the evening, many children begin to stay dry within six months of learning to use the potty.

Training at night takes longer as it also depends on how the body will retain urine for a long time. It can take months or years before the body of your child is sufficiently mature to stay dry at night. 10% of 7-year-olds and 5% of 10-year-olds are still allowed to wet the bed, the American Academy of Pediatrics says.

If he wants to sleep without diapers, let him go ahead. When he isn't ready for a couple of nights of this trial, bring him back in diapers without judgment.

Tell him that his body isn't ready for the next step and reassure him that he will be big enough to try again soon.

If your baby stays dry for 3 out of 5 nights, it's probably all right to make your official policy "all pants, all the time." Help him by restricting his drinking after 5 p.m. And get him up before you go to bed for a final bathroom ride. Don't worry if your child takes longer to stay dry overnight–night accidents are considered typical right up until school.

Ditch the diapers. When your child's ready to say goodbye to the slides, he's done a lot.

Recognize this and reinforce the pride of your child in its achievement by enabling it to give the remainders to a family with younger children or send them with the paint delivery service for the last time. You may also want to join it in a happy jig around the house and call it the "no more painting" dance.

WHAT SIGNS SHOW YOUR CHILD IS READY TO START POTTY TRAINING

The key to successful training begins when your son is physically interested, willing, and capable. While some kids are 18 months old, some may not be able to know until sometime after their third birthday. Many researchers suggest that boys remain a little longer in diapers than girls since they are usually more involved and are less likely to avoid using the potty.

It makes no sense to try to get a head start. If parents start potty training too early, it will possibly take longer. In other words, at the same time, you will arrive at your destination, regardless of when you start.

When your son is ready to begin potty training, concentrate on time. Stress or significant life changes, such as a new sibling or move, may complicate toilet training.

Ensure sure the routine of your child is well known. Wait until he is open to new ideas, and you can easily teach potty.

Check for signs of potty training to save both you and your child from time-consuming setbacks.

Is he yet ready?

First of all, before you even talk about potty training your boy, you have to make sure he's ready. Most babies are usually ready for potty training up to 18 months of age. Finally, in the 1960s, most babies were utterly potted.

Nowadays, however, the average age for potty training has doubled to nearly 36 months! A very different thing, for which we have to blame the modern diaper and its ultra-absorbing power.

Here are some clear signs that your kid is ready for potty training:

He has physical capacity for pulling pants up and down and squatting on potted pants.

He has regular, soft-shaped bowel movements.

He can interact with you-he can follow simple instructions.

Signs Your Kids Are Ready to Train

Boys dive on the potty a couple of seconds, and then go straight and pronounce the lesson over today. They may be less interested in learning how to go to a bathroom for many boys when they are right in their pants. And we don't concentrate on how to clean with boys, but we need to encourage them to reveal the penis when they go potty. If you've ever been sprayed as a small boy goes pee-pee, you're going to know why that's necessary.

If you trained other kids' potty, or this is your first one, you can find the potty you need to start can be a little different from girls to boys.

It's a little trickier for boys to shop for the right potty seat. Time will quickly become a huge mess if you're not looking for a potty with a splash barrier.

This guard stops you from being soaked or bogged down when it's time to go pee or poo. Since both can come out at the same time, it doesn't matter whether you teach your son to sit or stand when urinating, he's still sitting, and the splash guard is a must.

Boys ' moms and dads know you will be on your feet with male parents. The same goes for the potty training team. Boys ' incentives are bored. A tiny candy bar will have to be replaced tomorrow as a reward with a scoop of your favorite cereal.

Hold a stasis of potty incentives, like snacks, candy, books, toys, or even the prospect of visiting the children's museum, movies, or toy shop, at hand.

HOW TO HANDLE PROBLEM CHILDREN WHO REFUSE TO COOPERATE

Girls and boys will suffer accidents, even though they seem to have completed potty training. You're going to need a little longer to wear a change of clothes and wipes for your son than your daughter.

Most people don't want to feel dirty. We soon learn that if they don't stop doing what they want to do, they'll have soiled shoes and clothing. Accidents will occur, but girls must know as they understand the necessary steps of potty training.

Boys are more likely than girls to have injuries. Most don't mind if they walk around in their pants or soaking wet clothing or poops. Be prepared for these incidents at home or on your way, and get plenty of clean-up supplies and clothes ready for change.

Regardless of your gender, don't worry or scold your child when these incidents occur. Making potty training a negative experience at any stage will just bring a few steps back on your kids.

How do you handle incidents during potty training? How do you plan for potty exercise time? You can not place a clock on a child or postpone it with potty training. In their own time, they should complete toilet education, but gender should play a role.

While children of both sexes may receive potty training within a couple of days, the average time, a child is around three months for complete potty training. This is, when you have to use the toilet, you can ultimately remember it; you go to the toilet on your own, and you need little to no support to clean up. Girls typically complete all these potty training steps before boys.

Listen to your kids. Look for changes in actions that may trigger problems. You have to remember who they are with and where they are hanging out. You will be more confident by understanding where your child is. A big tip is to find the "Find my baby" program, one of the best ways for parents to keep an eye on the smartphone use and location of their baby. Aid can be provided if appropriate by this app on a smartphone or GPS watch.

Remember... as long as your child is healthy, take part in its developmental adventure. Combine compassion and firmness, and you will be delighted by the inevitable resolution of many issues.

Potty training tricks that made the process more comfortable can be tough. Here's how to make it a little more tolerable.

It is not surprising that potty training is one of the most challenging parts of raising a child. This is stressful. It's annoying (that a repetition warrant). The good thing is that once a child is ready to start potty training, parents can use a variety of tricks to motivate them. The majority of these are not new, and it's not necessary to reinvent the wheel thousands of years old, but it's worth listening to tips from parents with recent success. It's comforting if nothing else.

Here, then, are eight recommendations made by the parents, who recently made it through the potty training process with their health intact.

1. At least three dads have listed their experience with the episode of Daniel Tiger Potty Training. Titled "Daniel Goes

Potty," it reminds the children to STOP and go when they are to go. "We used it when we trained potty, and it helped him a lot," says Brian, Rockland County's two-daughter, New York. "It was instructive, indeed, but the most significant part was that it came from a character of whom he knew.

2. Using a "play-based" potty training program, Tot-on - the-Pot features a soft doll with its mini-toilet, a detailed kinship guide, 20 laminated activity cards, and a Tot on the Pot Board book. Dave Baldwin, the Fatherly publisher, told his daughter that the game was an outstanding "Partner-in- Poop." This not only offers a kid a chance to play potty with a doll, but the game-based rewards motivate children to conquer the toilet. New role-playing potty training games also help.

3. As potty boys learn, some fathers vowed by making potty training a target practice. It helped them conquer the commode by giving their son something to reach for — and having a game. You can buy or make your targets online. "I draw tissue paper boats and ducks, trying to sink the target," one father said. In any case, it is a useful technique for those who work not only on time but on precision and freedom.

4. This board book, in which Elmo teaches little children the art of potty, is not only written in the everyday, straightforward, dumb language but also has more than 30 interactive items to pull or move on every page. Most dads found out how helpful the book was in promoting and encouraging the notion of potty training in their potty activities.

5. Purchase the Travel Toilet Seat "We traveled quite a bit when our first girl was training in the potty, and this was the greatest support given how important coherence is," says Kevin, two dads in Louisville.

6. Take a choice and stick "Don't move between underwear and painting. We went to wear underwear all day (including nap

time) and pulling up at night (we call them underwear at night). The distinction is immense, and we do not use the toilet at any time of underwear, day or night, "one dad said. It could be a temptation to have a transitional phase when you start a potty training saga, from slides to underwear and back, depending on the time of the day. Yet this confuses a child, and his decision–even during naptime–to wear underwear all day helped his child with the program.

Potty training: overcoming five rising potty issues. Push the five most significant potty concerns away.

My first training was a breeze. Patience, perseverance, and a positive attitude. My daughter had a glimpse into the shop's Cinderella underpants and decided that it was time for her to use the pot as a big girl. She had been trained and sported her princess undies every day in about six weeks. So five years later,

I predicted the same quick turnaround when it was time to train my second daughter. But I was very shocked because my younger one didn't want fancy panties— or anything else relevant to potty training. Six months after her potty training began, I wasn't sure that she had caught up completely.

I have had two entirely different training experiences with my two children. And, as I discovered immediately, potty training is different for everyone.

But the outcome was the same: my children always learned to use the potty. Your child will also be on time. You should teach your child with patience, perseverance, and a positive attitude. That's not going to be issued along the way. According to Elizabeth Pantley, founder of the No-Cry Potty Training Solution (McGraw-Hill), more than 80 percent of children undergo reversals during toilet education. Here is a guide to solving several common pitfalls.

1: "If your kid doesn't want to use the pot, she's probably not ready," says Ari Brown, MD, co-author of Toddler 411 (Windsor Peak Press). And the first step is to make sure that your child is ready and knows everything about potty training. See if she is interested in the potty, stays dry for at least two hours a day, avoids playing, or hides as she fills the pressure or even asks for a clean one. If the signs are there, may the potty in the bathroom, store your pants, and work some potty journeys through your child's day. If not, the time will not yet be potty.

You may start to lay the groundwork by reading your kid's potty books, letting her play with a drinking and wet doll, or take her into the bathroom while using the toilet, even if she is not ready to start. However, if you don't care about the potty or start potty training and it's a power struggle, it may be time to leave for some time. "If your child is not ready and eager, there is no advantage to preparation," says Kristin Hannibal, MD, Clinical Director, General Academic Pediatrics Division, Pittsburgh Children's Hospital.

"Perhaps in a month or two, it's easier to go back to the slimmers and try again."

2: My kid only uses the potty when I put it. It is common for a kid to rely on mom's recollections in the early stages of the potty workout. After all, all his life he has spent peeing and pooping his slide anywhere he is needed. Dr.

Hannibal says that a little practice and experience will allow him to understand his body signs and to hit the potty in time. But if after a few weeks you still start every potty visit, you will be educated. Tell your kid that he is such a big boy that if he wants to go, he can get to the potty himself.

You can also add a winning scheme with a sticker or reward every time you go potty separately, says Dr. Hannibal. However, try to keep the rewards low. Julie Kelsey of

Germantown, Maryland, says, "We used Thomas Tank Engine trains to inspire our three-year-old son." "It worked, but it got pretty expensive!" While occasional accidents are natural, if your kid still does not get to the potty for a couple of more weeks— or has no interest in trying — he might not be ready for potty training.

3: My Child Can Pee but not Poop, in Potty, Check with your pediatrician to see if your child is blocked. In that case, a few changes to its diet–such as may fruit, vegetable and water intake, for example–are likely to do the trick. But if your kid won't use the potty but puddles in a painting without any problems, she will most likely be afraid. "It's terrifying to take toilets for many children," says Adiaha Spinks-Franklin, MD, a pediatrician at Texas Children's Hospital, Meyer Institute for Developmental Pediatrics in Houston.

"They can feel like they lose a part of their bodies when they pee," Spinks- Franklin says. "Or you may not like it if the waterfalls on the ground or if you're concerned about vomiting into the bathroom." Your child will need to solve this problem sometime, be careful with it. "By 2 1/2 she was just going to pee in a tub, I began potty training my daughter, Aila, who'd scream and keep her poop back," says Jennifer James, of Boone, Carolina of the North. "Eventually, we let her dick in a diaper until that glorious day, about six months after she hung into the toilet and figured out all was all right." To help the child conquer their anxiety, Dr. Brown suggests this incremental step-by-step technique. For a week or so, keep her dick in her drawing, but make her do it while she is sitting on the pot or the toilet. So, right before you put your child in the crib, cut out a hole with a pair of scissors and let her wear it while she uses the toilet. (We know it sounds nuts, but the diaper is still comfortable and healthy as the poop drops into the pot.) Once she's used the diaper hole for around one week, it'll be time for underwear!

4: My Child Only Goes Potty at Home Other children get used to their potted seats or toilet at home, and other bathrooms are typically leery. "All the toilets, particularly in public areas, are different," says Dr. Hannibal. "A bigger seat opening may make a child think that he would fall through, and an automatic toilet may be scary too." Help him get used to new bathrooms starting from one he's feeling comfortable, like that at the house of his best friend or Grandma's. Carry a pot with you when you need to go out in public or use a portable toilet seat cover to help him feel better.

5: My Child Is Potty Trained Throughout the day but Wakes Up Wet, Some parents think the dry night will go hand in hand with the dry day, but kids and pre-school children just can't stay dry at night. In reality, it's not uncommon for kids to wet the bed before the age of 7 with their tiny bladder and sound sleeping habits, Dr. Brown says. Place your child in a pair of panties or disposable training pants, and the whole family will sleep well (3-year-old Alex Ballad calls his painting "overnight underwear," according to his mum, Tricia from Bloomington, Illinois).

We know it's not easy, but try to keep your actions fun and optimistic— so your child can enjoy potty training. Be sure that you don't hurry her into preparation, discourage or be potty preparation the biggest challenge of her life. You're going to fight and deny if you do.

Here are a few ways to make the process simpler for you both: decorate the pot with one another. Write on it her name, or let it be embellished with stickers.

Enable her to choose her underwear or pants. She will be more inspired to smooth and dry her favorite characters or designs.

Encourage her, read, or let her blast as she sits on the potty.

Cheer her on when she's right. Create a funny potty song that you sing or dance happily in the bathroom together.

HOW TO GET DADS INVOLVED

How to get a father involved can be an exciting, daunting, rewarding, and frightening experience for mom, father, and children while you may all be gung ho about this idea, daddy maybe a little bit more reluctant to get involved. Training and reassurance will make a huge difference and hopefully allow this cycle for everybody to go smoothly.

Facilitate daddy to assist with this plan. You can ask him to read your kid's potty training book, so they both get to know the subject. Speak to your father about his hesitations and worries. Ease his worries with words of affirmation and simple explanations.

Remember the father of the many benefits of having a potty-trained boy. Second, the better your kid is taught potty, the better he does not have to wear the diaper bag on vacations. The money you save yourself from not having to buy clothes and towels is perfect and can be used for other items. It is no longer a plus to wipe dirty bottoms or deal with soiled diapers.

Explain the routine criteria and direct him through the process. If he's not familiar with the process, he may feel awkward. Talk him through a couple of potty training lessons, and he learns what to do. Tell him how to understand the potty dance signals and to get him quickly to the potty. Then give him the potty treatment: socks, on the toilet, falling, washing hands, happy potty dance, and a reward for staying. Remind him that your little one will sit on the potty chair several times a day for a few minutes each time. This should be done after meals and regularly all day long.

Ask your father to be a potty buddy and lead by example. This is especially important if you have a kid in school. The view and guidance of Papa are handy for your little one. Nonetheless, during the early stages, the website of the Mayo Clinic teaches your son how to sit down and pink before he learns the bowel movement stage. Daddy may just have to sit when your son accompanies him during this time if you two do not want to cleanse yourself of an inexperienced boy who can not target.

Speak to him in difficult times or have problem-solving when you're not around. Potty training can be an exciting, fun, stressful, and unfortunate period. Teach him how to manage potty accidents by reminding your child that it's okay and how to breathe deeply when the child wants to have uncooperative or stubborn moments.

Reward father also for his efforts. Potty training and all the mess that can come with it will make him in the knees a little weak. It may not be as healthy to him as it is to you, be quick to him. Give much praise if he participates willingly in the potty training process.

7 Ways Dads Can & Should Help With Tiny Training

Maybe the only time your child gets to sleep through the night is when you have slides. Potty training is a tradition to meet other parents, and neither is it shocking. After your child just ate some poop food, have you ever changed a diaper? It's not pretty. It is not beautiful. Yes, you do have to wash out their sometimes potty with potty training, but most of them are glad to make this deal. Women have historically been assigned post-diaper duties, but there are a variety of forms in which dads can and can assist with potty training.

My husband and I have a son, and I grew up with a friend, so I have a relatively small background in helping people to pull themselves into the toilet when I was designated driver at school. While I didn't have a (useful) background, I was eager to do my best. But I wasn't prepared to turn my son, now two years old, into a sport. Often it's like archery, others more of a crazy dance full of interpretation. That's why my partner was as supportive as it was to participate in the process. And see how dads can help with potty training.

1. Show & Tell It is quite boy-specific, but the basic argument applies universally. "Boys take toilet train a little longer probably because it is a mom who is doing all the teaching," says Potty Training Initiative. "It is often necessary that a boy shows him how their dad does it." After all, they work in the same pieces.

2. Talk About It One of the biggest obstacles you and your partner will face in this cycle is to keep things on the same page. Dr. Jan Faull, a parenting expert, told Pull-Ups that "contact is key in potty training. Speak to your partner daily about the progress and failures of your child so that the potty training strategy stays cohesive."

3. Note My partner is not a champion, and I'm still caught up in that relationship. If your child is going through a particularly difficult time where they avoid potty training, the process can quickly start to be seen as a race to complete. Take a step back and remind your friend that potty training does not mean who did it the quickest and when much like other childhood developmental milestones. Trust me; it eases the stress for those involved when you approach it differently.

4. According to potty training professionals Caroline Fertleman and Simon Cove, they proposed Parents that potty training will become more important to the child if the whole of a child's village (parents, professors, sitters, the family, etc.) provides encouragement and support.

5. But the simplest to do does not know how to use the toilet overnight. It can be exhausted if one parent is responsible for

keeping potty training enjoyable and exciting for the kid. The Baby Center says that imagination is essential for potty training. Whether it's food coloring to make the toilet colorful or using cereal for use, it's essential to keep your child involved. And when Dad is interested, it's easier to come up with ideas too.

6. Much like adults, children learn by continually learning and hearing knowledge. That is why fathers are so interested in the process. If your child sees both parents having the same conversation, they will catch on faster. It can be frustrating if you and your partner use the toilet, pee, or poo with different words. "The use of clear and accurate words will help your boy understand how to communicate about the toilet, according to the Mayo Clinic."

7. Grant You a break. There's a reason why people are watching the Walking Dead from the guard towers. You have to be alert and concentrated, and that won't happen if only one person is left. The same applies to potty training. According to What to Expect: The Toddler Years, "you can consider your child's signals clearer than they are. Watch for signs and ask where they are going to go." If your partner may have additional eyes and ears, the more likely you are of some potty chance.

TWELVE COMMON ISSUES WITH POTTY TRAINING

Working through traditional issues with potty training.

The transition from cloth to a pot is sometimes not smooth. Find more about these growing issues and what you can do about them with toilet training.

1. Your child is not conscious of the urination, despite knowing the need to move his bowels. That is normal. This is usual. For several months, some children will not achieve full bladder control despite learning to control bowel movements. Start the potty training of your child with this in mind.

2. Your child is trying to play with the feces. That's all because of his curiosity. You can stop it without upsetting him or her by just saying, "This isn't anything to play with."

3. Your son maintains that he sits to urinate. Most boys like to stay as they learn to go to the potty. Let him learn to urinate sitting down and tell him that the boys get up potty after he's mastered bladder control. He will handle it by himself, whether he watches the bathroom by his dad or by other male friends or relatives.

4. Your child refuses to go to the potty. Resistance may mean that training is not the right time to begin. Bring him to the potty anytime your child appears to have to urinate or have a bowel movement. Sit on the potty for just a few minutes at a time. Explain what you want to do. Be comfortable and relaxed. Don't demand if he objects strongly.

5. Your child is having accidents. Accidents happen. Accidents happen. Treat them gently and try not to get offended when they do. Punishment and scolding also cause children to feel bad, which may take more extended toilet training.

6. When she sees her stools flushed away, your child gets upset. Some kids believe their waste is part of their bodies, so it can be frightful and painful for them to understand. Explain the function of body waste and the need for the body to eliminate it.

7. Your child is afraid to be pulled into the toilet. Many children are fearful that it is sucked into the toilet when it's flushed. Let him or her flush pieces of toilet paper to give your child a sense of control. This will be raising fear of the running water sound and the sight of objects that vanish.

8. Your child is bowel movement or urinates directly after the toilet is removed. This also occurs early in the potty workout. Your child can need time to learn how to relax the bowel and bladder control muscles. If this happens a lot, your child might not be ready to learn.

9. Your child demands a diaper if there are a bowel movement and stands in a particular position to defecate. This means that she is physically ready to be taught but not emotionally. Alternatively, thank your child for understanding bowel signs instead of viewing them as a failure. Say that while wearing a diaper, he or she has bowel movements in the bathroom.

10. Your child urinates during the night. For other kids, your kid would probably take a little longer for nap and night toilet training. Encourage your child to use the potty right before he goes to bed and when he wakes up. Tell her that he can either go alone or call you to help him if he wakes up in the middle of the night and wants to use the bathroom.

11. Your child is only confident with a specific person to go to the potty. That is normal. This is usual. When your child goes with you only, step by step, remove from the process. For starters, provide support to undress your child or to take your child to the bathroom. Wait outside the entrance, however.

12. Your child returns to her art days. Something that induces stress in children may lead them to revert to an earlier stage of growth, mainly if the change is recently made. Stressors include a child's disease or a relative's disease, a new baby in the home, a shift from bed to bed, or moving to a new home. Give it time, and it's going to happen.

WHAT TO DEAL WITH THE REGRESSION OF POTTY TRAINING

Does a potty kid unexpectedly experience accidents? Figure out why there is a potty regression— and how to avoid it.

Everything is going well: your little boy appears to have mastered potty training, and you think you have done good luck with the diapers. But then he begins to have injuries all of a sudden, and you wonder what went wrong.

We'll explain why a child can take a couple of steps backward when it comes to potty training.

Get more potty training tips

A child plays with toilet paper. Make sure it is real that many children have a potty regression — it's natural. But ask yourself if your child was potty at first. "It's really common in the early days, months, or even years of potty training with occasional failures," said Scott J. Goldstein, MD, Northwest Children's Practice pediatrician, Chicago. "Just note that a potty kid who is disciplined would like to go to the potty. Thus, a child who is in many accidents each day and doesn't seem to care [for them] just should not be called' potty training.' If he did, continue to try ways to get back on track. If not, speak to your doctor if she feels your child might be ready.

Do not overreact. When an incident happens to your child, do not express disappointment; this could make your child upset, which in effect could lead to more potty issues. "To do whatever you can to be optimistic is to be disappointed by the accidents and diapers triggered by the backward toilet regression," says Wendy Sue Swanson, M.D., Parents ' advocate and pediatrician at the Seattle Children's Hospital. If you see that your child is healthy, clap, and cheer. If not, just stay unconvinced and say, "Oops. You have had an accident. Let's go sit on the potty." Remember to be optimistic and never yell at or scold your kid. "You wish your kids were motivated and not afraid they would get punished if they made a mistake," says Lisa Asta, MD, University of California Clinical Professor of Pediatrics, San Francisco. **Resolve the root causes.** If you don't fix the exact issue, you can not avoid the reverse. Mark Wolraich, MD, Head of the Development and Behavioral Pediatrics Department of the University of Oklahoma's Centre, and Director of the Child Studies Centre, says, "It's helping the child return to its position to understand the causes for the regression. Most children, for example, tend to have incidents in adjustment periods that may trigger stress, like beginning a new school or adopting a new sibling. The chances are that once your lives are settled, your child can again master potty training. Yet even though your child does it without injuries during the day, she will still have malfunctions at night. "Most children aren't dry at night years after daytime are dry," says Dr. Goldstein. "Nighttime and naptime management are very different from the daytime." Health complications can also lead to a decline in potty training, which is normal. When a child has trouble with bowel movement, she should clear the potty entirely to prevent pressing and straining. Be sure your child gets enough water and food, but when she is scared of pooping, playing games, or reading books with her while she is sitting on the toilet and making it fun.

Sometimes, injuries occur when a child's play or activity is too fun and simply does not want to avoid running to the toilet. To overcome this the problem, clarify that you often fail to use potty and reassure your kid that she is still "a great person," says Dr. Goldstein. Then, at home, take her to the potty every couple of hours and encourage her teachers to make sure that she goes to the potty. Clear positive reassurance and potty reminders will help your child get back on track.' Encourage your child to at least use the potty when she wakes up first, before meals, before bedtime, and just before you leave.

Try the rewards— to a degree. Offer a few incentives to stay dry, particularly if you have trained him for the first time. Develop a sticker chart and give a sticker to your child every day he has no accident. You can compensate him for several good days in a row, such as a trip to the ice cream shop or a small gift, or less traditional incentives such as offering ten extra minutes of bedtime reading or enabling him to see a short film at breakfast. Nonetheless, bear in mind that incentives do not work for every child and can cause as much fear in certain situations as punishments can do. That's why your words are always the best rewards: "You're such a smart kid!" or "You're so confident" often can be the best motivation.

POTTY PROBLEMS: 4 SOLUTIONS TO YOUR TOILET PROBLEM

Your child may have diapers, but toilet training is not over. Using our suggestions to cure the blues in your children's bathroom.

It was a happy day when I taught my oldest boy. For me, it didn't mean the mess of diapers anymore. To him, it represented the status of a big boy.

However, then came our mega-mart ride— the public bathroom. My usually trustworthy son entered the stall and bolted out quickly. Our problem? Our problem? Everywhere the bane of little children: the dreaded self-flush toilet.

(My son poorly identified the red sensor as "the blind eye" for years.) You may think that you are facing past bathroom issues as soon as your children have been certified "officially qualified toilet." Yet there are other challenges, even for a kid who is a potty pro. "Learning to use a bathroom requires a variety of processes, but parents may encourage their children to master the bathroom by keeping calm and encouraging," says Edward Christophersen, Ph.D., Children's Mercy Hospital clinician in Kansas, Missouri.

Toilet problems:

Wetting Incidents: That usually occurs when a child is not over-enthusiastic. She has a full bladder, and she's psyched so much about something ("A party pony!") she can't contain herself and pees on her pants. A kid may have accidents even if it is kept in chronic conditions, said Steve J. Hodges, M.D., professor of pediatric urology at the Baptist Medical Center at

Wake Forest University, Winston-Salem, North Carolina. "The bladder is like every other muscle," he says. "While you've been walking the potty all day, every day, you're constantly squeezing your bladder." It's thickening your muscles and making your bladder smaller. It will begin to contract with less notice and more force very soon— and your child will end up with water pants.

The remedy is to ensure that she frequently goes to the toilet. Children of this era do not always know that they have to go before it's too late. You may not have to follow her every 10 minutes to the toilet, but know how much she went last time (and how much she was forced to drink). When she grows older, she becomes more in line with the rhythm of her body.

Public bathrooms: Going to the bathroom is a private experience, which makes it common for children to murmur about a busy, noisy toilet— and often dumb— face it. Your kid would never want to go potty, but by planning ahead and by looking at you using public toilets, whether at church or store, you will make it simpler.

Make a few visits when he doesn't have to go, says Lawrence Balter, Ph.D., a psychologist in New York City, to help him feel comfortable with the process. When he is scared of different noisy sounds, just point them out politely. Say, "Yeah, look. It's loud when you're pressing the button and breathing in the air to dry your face." If you stop next time, ask if he can press it.

As for the sensor toilets? Any child may be frightened by a surprising flush that refuses to use one ever again. The same approach is suggested by Dr.

Balter. "Well when he's using the toilet, just place it in front of him, and calmly say to him,' You don't even have to push anything, and the toilet flush the paper for us.'" Clever moms bring in their pockets a few post-it notes.

Hold one over the "blinky eye," and it won't blow until your kid needs it so he can pee comfortably.

Wiping cleaning is easy for most children to deal with after urination, but it's another story after a bowel movement. "Many 3-and4-year-olds have little energy or ability to do the job properly," Dr. Christophersen says. "Children typically need to be at least five to do this properly." But you can encourage your child to get it right now.

The best way to do so is to teach the process of "wiping, looking, and falling." Make sure to explain how you firmly wipe the tissue and place it in the toilet. Remind her that the cycle must be repeated before the tissue is clean and thoroughly washed by hand. Keep it clear and truthful, and skip any additional comment if it's messy. After you have taught her how to clean once or twice, hand the job over to her, but test your own afterward. If your child is a neatnik, she may not even want to try it, but she will remain firm.

This ability must be learned by pre-school students.

Constipation, Your child may get constipated because he wants not to go or because it could be his diet or a scarcity of fluids that backs him up.

Nevertheless, it can become a vicious cycle: if he doesn't go a while, he becomes harder and more frustrating–and that doesn't make him want to. "For a child, it is important to eat plenty of fiber and when he is encouraged to go," Dr. Hodges says. Yet bathroom breaks are not high on the priority list of any child. He'd just prefer to keep it in and continue to play with his mates.

You can't push him into the toilet, and certainly don't want to turn the situation into a power battle that you all will lose. "The inevitable desire to go to get him to the bathroom happens in the morning or after a meal," says Hodges. Provide high-fiber foods, such as wheat pasta, black beans, and apples. Speak to your doctor about whether it would be good to give your child a stool softener like Miralax. When his constipation–or some other potty condition–seems to be a chronic condition, the doctor will want to see to it that there are no other issues.

HOW DO YOU START POTTY TRAINING? SIX WORST MISTAKES PARENTS MAKE DURING 3-DAY POTTY TRAINING.

Can you practice at night at the same time? Below are a few things that are normal and do not.

So you're able to start potty exercise, but aren't you sure whether you want to try a three-day approach or something gradual? We asked Janice Heard, a Calgary community pediatrician, what that mistakes parents have to make as they try to improve their baby's toilet training. (Hint, some of her' don'ts' are actually in some three-day approaches listed as' must-dos.')

1. "I have parents who swear to their 18-month-old baby who has a toilet training and there are real exceptions, such as we often see 8-month-old babies walking that's early, but it does happen," Heard says. Nevertheless, in most instances, she says the parents train themselves. "The caregiver senses the movements and signals of the infant and helps them get to the toilet on time," she says. It's all right if your kid keeps your bladder reasonably full, so you're all right with a lot of hands-on potty time every time, so it could be a concern if you suggest you leave it for a day or a babysitter with the grandparents for an evening. Many carers will not be able to hold the network up, so it can be stressful for everybody, says Heard. The majority of children are between two and four years old until they can be educated consistently in the bathroom, she said.

2. "It is not unusual for children to have blood levels for several months until they can have complete control of their bowels," Heard says. "One of the risks is that a child can get very swept away." This happens when a child has some unfortunate encounters with the potty and then develops a fear of it. When you have no choice of using your diaper, you can want to remain in your poo for days. "And it's frustrating when they eventually go. This increases the dimension of fear and can become a vicious cycle, "she says. Consult your doctor if your child is frequently constipated and in pain.

3. Not using constructive potty talk. Use derogatory terms for the poo and pee of your infant, including "bad" or "stinky," is validated by some of the three- day approaches we tested, like 3-day Lora Jensen potty training, but it is a mistake, said Heard, which can affect your self-esteem. "Children respond to appreciation, positive reinforcement and loving encouragement," she says. "Of course, you may be able to get them to do what you want to by being aggressive or furious, but that's a fearful answer." And if kids are ever disciplined for an incident, it can adversely affect the relationship between their parents and their children, Heard said. "Never should children be disciplined for anything for which they have no full control," she says. It helps parents, if possible, to avoid disappointment or annoyance. "The facial expression can be counterproductive, like' oh no, not again.'"

4. Doing' night exercise' is due to a maturation delay in the brain, whereby children need longer to learn to regulate their bladder during the night. "It's beyond their influence," Heard says. She advises that you use overnight exercise pants and waterproof mattress clothes before your child stays on her bladder while she sleeps. "About

10% of children also wet their beds at the age of eight, which is where we begin to interfere medically," Heard says. Unless a medical condition is present, all children can eventually catch it — no real "training" is required at night.

5. So many incentives give children standing in front of a toilet. Do you try three days of potty training?"Kids don't even need a potty smartie," Heard says. After all, for any trip to the bathroom, they do not continue to collect candies until training is over. Lobbying is satisfying enough for most children, she says. When your child is 3.5 or 4, and you just believe they need extra support, then get the treatments done. "But it's not something that I suggest, to begin with," she says.

6. If you contradict your training with the parents of your child, you should try to have their child trained as soon as possible so that they develop an inaccurate understanding of the abilities of their child. "They misunderstand that they should catch their child every growing time they pee and keep it out of pains, confusing it with real growth," says Heard. This can make them feel like a failure if parents do not meet their child in time— or the little man has an accident at the home of the grandmother or the babysitter. "People who are in a hurricane end up with more injuries and more stressful moments, and this is not a healthy way to be with your kids," Heard said.

5 HARD FACTS ABOUT POTTY TRAINING

Potty Training is a lousy business, and even because you have a strategy, this does not guarantee your children's success in the bathroom.

Well-thought-out potty training plans can trick parents into a false sense of health. Given the implied messages sent by adorable sticker map, candy rewards, hype "No-Pants Cycle" and cheerful DVDs, the potty training process is rarely straightforward and nearly invariably tall. The truth of potty education is very far away from sanitized explanations of parenting books that contain lovely euphemisms. Simply put, things get wild. Yet parents are better prepared for this inevitability.

Faced with the blunt reality about potty training early on, parents should brace themselves for gross contingencies and speak frankly about their concerns. This also sets expectations and stops parents from believing that they are doing anything wrong. They're not in all probability. It's just a robust operation.

1: Parents: Don't know whether parents will be desperate to avoid changing clothes. We might also face daycare demands or pre-school deadlines. Yet if a child is not ready for potty training, the cycle will fail. This is always in the best interest of all to wait.

To be effective and relatively painless in potty training, a child must demonstrate an interest in using the toilet. And there are also subtle signals, like hiding behind a sofa in the pull-ups, or arguing with parents while sitting in the toilet. A child is less likely to ask for the toilet, but it is not out of the realm of possibility.

But, when parents pressure a child into potty training, children are very freaked. They may be afraid of the process, become stubborn, and eventually drag out the potty workout. This may cause a parent to be angry and cause the child to be guilty. This is a horrific downward spiral.

2   Kids learn how to use the Potty by looking at their parents. Some parents can realize that their private lives have been demolished; their second child may be born at the door of the bathroom. And while it's a bushman to make a child look at a single poop time, it allows them to understand the bathroom cycle. No.

Children learn, by watching what their parents do, to communicate with the environment. If the bathroom is a robustly guarded secret, children near the potty age of training may be very wary of using the potty. After all, when a parent goes behind a locked door into the bathroom, then it must be a massive, intimidating operation.

On the other hand, children will test how the mechanism works if parents have an open door policy. This makes them realize that being picky isn't a big deal. Big people do it. Small people do it. And there is no specific magic or mystery about people flushing material inside.

3. Children's Potty Training Will Poop and Pee happen on the carpet. Often a kid can't get in time to the place. Often they wake up early. Anyway, the excrement and urine will be outside the toilet. Parents need to become used to it.

This reality is particularly harsh for parents who are using the "no-pants" system, which only gives children a couple of days off. Advertising This can work, but it's a good idea to have a few extra towel rolls and a cleaner floor because a mess is practically guaranteed.

4. Potty Training Regressions. Even when parents believe their kid has the entire situation of potty training, their kid starts moisture his pants again. This turn of events is not uncommon and can occur as it goes from simple diversion to diet to a routine slip.

The critical thing to remember for parents is to stay calm. The higher a parent becomes, the more resistant a child can become to potty training. The trick is to stay optimistic, to stick to the plan, and to keep the child underwear.

Alert. If a parent is particularly worried about regression. You should speak to a doctor. A medical professional can help assess what the problem is so that the parent can prevent wild speculation and throw plans into confusion. 5: Training children how to wipe. Tough Potty is a training kid who cannot wipe themselves properly. The practice is needed. Yet not just self-directed work. Wiping is part of a potty routine that parents may need the most because it is not as easy as pooping or peeing in a tube.

Since wiping can be challenging to understand, parents may want to wipe their safety wipes. You should also expect to see dirty underwear until your child gets used to the wiping process. This is just the way it goes.

There are so many reasons why you want to train your child as a potty as early as possible. The risk of early potty training your son. You want to stop buying diapers; they're costly and harmful to the climate. You want your kid to be in front of the game. There is no brainer for early potty training.

Nonetheless, the reasons why your child needs to train potty early sound ridiculous in contrast with the severity of the reasons you should not.

This is unfair to place children under three years old in a position that makes them entirely liable for their toilet behavior, says Dr. Steve Hodges, M.D., from BedwettingAndAccidents.com.

HOW WOULD EARLY POTTY TRAINING

POSSIBLY GO WRONG?

If it comes to early potty training, children should be taught potty long before the age of three, but are they? If you use the potty, it can lead to many health issues if you do it poorly.

Dr. Hodges believes that out of the approximately 100 children he sees in his clinic every week, about half were potty trained before the age of three and that they are so-called "dysfunctional vacuums," which cause urinary tract infections, weathering, and sudden occurrence (regression). When a child has persistent diarrhea, the rectum consists of a mass that fills the space that the bladder uses to contain urine. The nerves may become agitated by mass and cause irregular bladder contractions. Such unwanted contractions, combined with the lack of urine capacity, often cause urination and accidents.

It's getting even stressful. This poo build-up in the rectum produces lots of bacteria. And that bacteria are very likely to creep through the bladder and trigger bladder infections in younger ones, mainly if they are prone to pee too.

You're not alone when you're cringing about all of this pee and poop talk. Many parents conclude that potty training issues are very common and do not bother to report them to their pediatricians. However, it must be addressed.

Recent studies have shown that avoiding holding habits and abnormal voiding is crucial to the prevention of injuries, bedwetting, and bladder infections, including those reported by the National Center for Biotechnology Knowledge.

How are these things related to early training?

The explanation that little ones who train potty even at the age of 2 have more issues than children who wait until the age of 3 are not mature enough to determine themselves when they will pick and pound. You also don't know the value of proper elimination if you experience the urge and elimination entirely. Dr. Hodges says that the bladder shrinks every year while urine is retained, thereby making it more overactive.

What are you going to do?

Look for signs that your child is ready for the potty train, such as WebMD.com signs.

Tell your child every two hours to use the toilet. Don't ask. You're just too busy to have fun, so keep it as long as possible. This is a risky habit that strengthens the bladder so that the child is desensitized to feeling full, and the bladder leaves on its own.

Don't bow to the strain of the peer. If a school or daycare provider advises you that your child needs potty training before attending, find a different provider.

Remind them to "get all out" before they exit the bathroom.

You may be one of those lucky parents whose child "gets" it right from the bat. Right, maybe your child is two years old. But know that you're not alone for parents who also have problems in teaching potty. Probably, you're in the majority.

You wouldn't trust a boy to brush his teeth every night correctly, so you shouldn't trust a boy to know how to remove it every night. Remember, early potty training will expand your duty to track your bathroom activities closely. **Further Potty training resources: risks of early training**

The correlation between the age of toilet training and dysfunctional validation. Every parent knew the one thing I wish before they began potty training.

When helping children (and parents) achieve some milestone, I also speak about encouragement. What would inspire a child to pursue and excel in the next milestone? This is also the secret to any new ability.

The cotton training pants were the answer when it came to potty training for us. If a child does not feel wet, he is not inspired to learn the strategies required to prevent this discomfort. If life stays the same for them and a junk pair or training pant takes the moisture away, and they look as they always do, what's the fuss?

When you can concentrate your attention on potty exercises and train your child to adopt cotton pants regularly, gently, and motivated, such pants are only "double stuffing" underwear and can continue to be worn until a kid grows up for the bad shots in the bathroom, long carriages or uncooperative straps or snaps.

Potty training is not the scariest skill a parent will teach his boy! Confide in me; driving is the most frightening thing your child will ever do!

Why parents procrastinate when training potty

The short answer. Before making single clothes, parents were highly motivated to get their children out of clothes and to avoid the endless process of transition, purge, and washing.

Parents grabbed the opportunity at the first indication of any interest and led their child down the road to potty independence! These symptoms typically started to appear around 15-18 months if the kid had older siblings much earlier.

So why are kids not good in potty training until 30–40 months now. And they can, again. Parents believe that their child is not old enough when signs begin to appear at 18 months and ignore healthy development. I can't tell you how many parents of the 3-year-old who are planning for a kindergarten school tell me that "he was so interested a year ago now that it's time for him not to look out on the potty." Accessible slides are comfortable and do not include the aggressive laundry process that eliminates incentives from the parent, and we are conditioned to believe that children must be able to go to a nursery school. All of these things are real, but you don't want to wait for it right before kindergarten school.

In reality, any pre-school teacher would tell you that potty accidents for children who are barely educated before they go to kindergarten are frequently avoided. Why can a child or its peers excel in the foundations of learning and socialization when potty accidents still interrupt them?

The Help-A-Potty-Mess, quote from our friend Happy, "The world is a Potty Mess!"But it must not be. Late in 18 months, the American Academy of Pediatrics recommends safe and effective potty training. Only think about all the right things: a well-trained preschooler, hundreds of about $in the monthly savings, and room for a kid who doesn't have a blast!

Parents Should not postpone their child's potty training. Before beginning your child's potty training, you will expect various outlets to provide details on this process. Parenting newspapers, family, friends, and experts are some of the outlets. There are several approaches and recommendations available to support this mission. In the first place, a curriculum appropriate for you and your child must be chosen. When you have two children, it is not compulsory for one approach to work with both children. You might have to use a program for one child and a completely different program for another child.

Some parents typically don't want to train their children until they hit the age of two. You are waiting for the moment when your child speaks the words of toiletries.

On the other hand, some children can learn at this age quickly, and others create difficulties because when a child turns two, they want to do everything that they want to do. When you say, "It's time to go potty," they generally refuse because they don't want to carry out such an operation. Another thing that will panic the trainer that the child can begin to weep before his wishes are fulfilled.

When the child grows up, he does a lot of work, and it is difficult to persuade them to stay on the potty for a long time. A child will begin to play instead of taking the time to pause and use the potty.

One of the main disadvantages of late potty training is that children are usually recognized by pre-schools, who are entirely eligible for potty. Due to this error, children can not be admitted to kindergarten on time, which eventually is an obstacle to their entire education career.

Parents should recognize their child's signs associated with toilet activities and be the only adult who can contribute substantially to a child's potty training. Parents should also be vigilant and not prolong their child's potty training.

THE JOY OF POTTY BOYS LEARNING!

At least the boys have more steps in the overall potty exercise. In the absence of these steps in a particular order, small boys that pee in your engagement party (true story) on your sister's feet.

It is also recommended to encourage small boys to follow their example for dads or other trusted people. But when you're a single woman, what do you do?

The first step is the same for boys and girls in potty training. All should begin training by sitting down!

The "sit-training" portion ensures trust, consistency, and a better target. Before a little boy can confidently and regularly take this measure, he will not go on.

Therefore, whether they use the bowl, the toilet, or wherever they are, they must enter the toilet comfortably and have the right balance.

When you are practicing, it can be helpful to offer young boys goals that they can see. Floating cereals are mostly used by parents and items that use projected lights, and all kinds of fun variants are now available.

You also hear that boys are tougher, that's not my experience, but that each child is different. My advice is to start recognizing the symptoms at 18 months. Make sure you set an example for your boy, pick the process you want, and make it an adventure!

Child Training Tips: Seven Potty Training Tips

Some young people refuse to advertise their products, keep their own, and endure all attempts to train them potty. If you're annoyed that you only buy diapers and you don't use the pottery chair, read on.

Later toilet training, such as slow walking, can be the natural developmental pattern of your child and can be shared with mom and dad while you are in school. The nerves and muscles involved in potty training may still not be mature. Suspect this cause if your child is in certain developmental milestones at the late end of normal. Some children are on a three-year path through bowel and bladder school. If you and your child have made little progress, find these potty training tips and tools in addition to consulting your baby's doctor:

1. Find Medical Reasons. A child does not perform any dangerous bodily act. Constipation is painful and also induces tiny tears in the rectum as the infant strains, thereby restricting the infant to its intestine and continuing a painful process. Suspect that if your child squats, grunts and grimaces, but does not produce anything. A soft stool breakfast (fresh fruit, whole-grain cereal rich in fiber, and plenty of fluids all day long) will open the day to resistant small bottoms.

   Bottom food allergy burning may be another culprit. Look for the allergic ring telltale and the raw anus patch. High-acid foods such as citrus fruits and foodstuffs containing lactic acid are typical criminals, including dairy products. Diarrhea stools can also temporarily impede bowel function during flu or after the use of antibiotics.

2. Don't move too hard; too soon, Potty training may have started too early, or a teacher and pupil can clash at a negative period. Tell yourself what could or could not happen in the life of your baby that makes it reluctant. Consider backing the following emotional slumps for a while that could delay training: Does the baby experience a depressive period in which he is not receptive to something new?

Is the situation troubling in the household: a new baby, a big relocation, household tension, longer working hours, a return to jobs, or a disease? Is your child furious? Anger shuts down all physiological processes, especially toilets.

3. Rewards work. Make a friendly game of potty training. Place a toilet sticker diagram. He gets a sticker every time he goes potty on his own. He gets a generous reward after a few stickers. Some tips for the right incentives include eating small meals, working on new toys, or bringing two bottles of coin into the toilet. Each time he walks by himself (even with support and encouragement), let him take a coin out of his full jar and place it in his jar. Sure he can go to the potty regularly to get more money, but it's cheaper than diapers.

4. Dump the diapers. Potty fitness advice from our family: It's all right to lie a little. Some children won't be educated in the toilet until their diapers are giving up. One day just announces: "The store has no diapers left" or "The diapers all are gone." Let him run around with just a long shirt (if it's warm enough) and bare-bottomed. Or, fortune goes bare-bottomed in the house. (You'll save what you spend on carpet cleaning on the slide.) Going bare-bottomed allows him to assume greater responsibility for his body functions.

5. The best time for a bowel movement is around 20 minutes after a meal. Set a toilet routine Enable your son to sit on a pot after a meal-preferably after breakfast, so he enters a regular toilet routine.

6. If your 3-year-old has "activities" that you believe are due to laziness, inattention, or just pretending to be a kid again, let him share the burden of cleaning up, not punctually, but respectfully. Tell him how to wash his pants and then hamper them to be cleaned. Expect older children to return during a miserable time, during a disruption in the family, or shortly

after a new sibling arrives. If you believe he is old enough to take responsibility for his body functions, briefly forget the pant soiling, telling him that if he decides to walk in his pants uncomfortably, this is his decision. You want him to get the message that this is his, not yours. If you believe he stains his pants so that you deserve extra attention (bottom cleaning is a great deal of hands-on attention), increase your constructive attention, even for cleanups. Give him particular tasks with one parent around the house and special one-on-one trips. You want to tell him that you pay more attention to the right actions than to negative behavior.

7. Realize that it can be a question of control. It can be the way your child can influence one part of his life you can not influence. If you keep your kidneys in certain places firmly (choice of clothes, sweets, pastimes, etc.), don't be shocked if you get stuck there. It may be the only way he knows how to live a little longer. This might be the time to close the potty deck for a few weeks or months to settle for your kid, to have fun, and reinforce the connection. If your child is emotionally depressed already and has low self-esteem, be careful not to say that the worth of your child depends on success. This first number in parenting, whether in toilet training or the Little League, is a good strikeout. The task of the caregiver in toilet training is to facilitate: Set the conditions for the child to go smoother. The rest belongs to the dad.

6 Ways You Can Hemming Your Kid's Potty Training Progress

The first thing I will remember about your kid's potty training is that he or she is a kid. If you have ever encountered another parent attempting to teach their child unsuccessfully to go to the potty, it may have been challenging to say who is who.

You, of course, are smarter than this, but only if-here are six ways you can hinder the success of your child's potty training.

Your Face says, "You've failed," "I am angry with you," and "I'm disappointed, again." You don't have to pronounce a word because these emotions are written on your face. Your child reads your face and knows what you think precisely. They don't miss much.

You get disappointed in yourself because, well, someone special to you was disappointed. You know they failed again, so maybe next time they won't try too hard. That is how potty training is losing, losing condition quickly.

Each time, no matter how complicated, do your hardest to cover up the feelings of wrath and frustration and then SAY the contrary.

Mom Do All Training, Of course, moms usually get the most from potty training incidents and complaints, but if your child is a boy, then it's a chance for dad to get big-time involved. A small (and big) boy doesn't want anything but to please his dad, so this is an excellent chance to do so.

Sit next to the toilet his potty, so that he and dad can "do their jobs" together. When it's effective, Dad's "excellent job! "And the universe would say to him high five. Nor is it wrong to sit together without success, because it will give your son a good example. Maybe add a book or pretend to complete the image by mobile phone.

This is so easy to do when one step forward and two steps back appear to carry you. Your child has another accident, just as you think things are improving. Do not think you need to go backward and change what you are doing if you have switched from painting pants to training pants. Hang in there.

Be routine-compatible. Encourage your child to sit right before bed on the potty or toilet in the morning and when he or she leaves home. This routine will finally pay off.

Often you just need to loosen it, but keep it out of the sight of the little ears of your kid. They are even though you don't think they're listening. It is much worse than the emotions on your neck. Mostly you tell someone else how sad you are, how upset you are, how unintelligent you are, that they don't know.

Punishment doesn't work, so it doesn't work either.

Who cares how early your neighbor's child has learned to regulate his body functions? It isn't a rivalry between you and other people. It's not a game where the winner and the loser are present. It is a teacher and tutor learning cycle. This requires patience. If they don't seem to advance, try another tactic or return for a while and note, this isn't about you!

Being the Poop Police Instead of being the parent who reports mistakes, focus on any little success, and enjoy each of them entirely. Laughter is a way to make things simpler, and children sure like to laugh.

Initiate a "silly dance" and do it when useful. Hold a star calendar for those in the family to focus on the progress every day. Ignore some bad days. Find a way of celebrating a positive development that will make both your child and you smile and laugh.

All things are going to pass, and so it is.

Potty Boys Literally!

Potty boys carry on a completely different sense and method than potty girls. For example, boys usually begin at a later age than girls do, but experts can not understand why.

Potty boys ' training typically begins at the age of 24-36 months; this varies between kids.

Boys appear to have more accidents and urinate more often at night than girls do, and it takes a little more work for boys to keep them dry.

Make sure your kid doesn't offer any late-night fluids about 1 hour before going to sleep. This gives him the ability to remove everything in his system before he goes to his room.

Before starting a kid's potting training, you have to decide if he's ready by showing you that he's able to sustain a dryness most every night.

If you think he's set, go out and buy a dozen or so clothes pants; these are the ones that he will wear in the daytime. Keep the portable slides handy for potty training at night. Understand that injuries can occur; this is part of the learning process.

When your boy has an accident, don't show disgust! Instead, he acknowledged an error empathically and lovingly and encouraged him to do better next time.

When potty trainers repeat their affirmation of expectations during their training, while displaying compassion, they have a substantial advantage over the average person who is irritated and upset. As a result; you can train your boy much faster and more effectively!

HOW TO DO A SUCCESSFUL 3-DAY POTTY TRAINING

Potty training is an integral part of parenthood. Although this can be difficult, potty training is not as hard as some parents would think. It can be completed only in 3 days! Did your eyebrows lift this statement? Do you doubt the notion of potty training for three days and think it's either a joke or a jerk?

Early planning is also essential for the big day. For example, you can buy potty and some trainers and undies two weeks before the actual training begins. It would also help if the app is activated and your child can play with it.

The idea is to make your kid feel confident with the potty. Your practice for your pre-potty training day ends the night before the first session. Know that evening; your kid will be a big day tomorrow, as he/she will be a big boy/girl. During the entire training cycle, there should be no disruptions. Make sure your plan is transparent so that you can completely commit your baby to train for three days.

Place the potty in an accessible area and ensure that all other resources are ready on the training day itself.

Training

It takes a lot of concentration, discipline, and dedication to excel in your child's potty training. Yeah, it can be tough; but that doesn't mean it can't be. Here are the ways to make it effective: welcome the day of your child with a smile, and tell him/her cheerfully that he/she will pin and pick on the potty starting today. Place the fresh undies on it. Immediately afterward, urge him/her to drink a big glass of milk or water to avoid peeing. Set a timer and try to place your child every 15 minutes on the potty.

In addition to being concentrated, you should also anticipate accidents. Patiently remind your child after any mistake to pee or poop on the potty. Don't make your child stressed. Praise him for every performance. For every achievement.

Also, specific treatments such as stickers or candies may produce more positive outcomes. Let your child know with every achievement that he/she does a beautiful job and that you are pleased with it.

The preparation will take place all day long. At night, sleep pants are recommended.

Only keep doing what you did on the first day. Depending on your child's reaction to training, you may make some time interval adjustments. For example, every 30 minutes instead of 15, you can grow your child on the potty.

The last day of training is incredibly significant because it determines the quality of your child's training. You should remove the use of a timer this day. Only ask your child if he/she needs to choose. If appropriate, put your little one on the potty.

There you have it; your child's 3-day potty training. This training is sure to be useful if you have enough concentration and patience.

Suggestions Useful for Potty Training Boys

The time spent on potty training boys in most situations is much harder, and it takes longer than girls do. So at the start, I want to stress my recommendations that a boy's parents should have patience. It's best to be calm, take time, and step along with the toilet only when you see the baby kid is ready for the new work.

Potty kids are a little sick of parents and do not lose. Parents who have a female baby earlier should be cautious not to try to do the same when their second child is a boy.

The best thing will be to praise your baby when he completed the operation. In most situations, you will find that your baby boy is demanding a pot after proper toilet training and has shown signs of removing his diaper because he wants to change it. Again there is a range of fantastic items on the market designed to make the entire potty training phase a fun and adventure for kids.

As a child's parents, you must give your baby boy such a potty that encourages him to use it. Introduce the act of blowing the potty in front of your boy so that it can encourage the boy, and he can only be persuaded to come out of the cloth and to do the act. The small boys ' parents benefit from not using disposable diapers but using tissue diapers.

Friends also help a lot and are also very good for potty kids. There is also a range of helpful books for suggestions for potty training boys. So you may buy these books if necessary and complement the potty training for boys.

Other beautiful items can also be useful for parents.

POTTY TRAINING DISCREPANCIES BETWEEN BOYS AND GIRLS

There is a big difference between potty boys and girls. One common mistake parents make to educate their child without worrying about how sex works. Your child's biological features play a significant role in the potty training process. Furthermore, studies have shown that girls appear to learn faster than boys in most situations.

There is a gender gap between boys and girls when it comes to potty training. While some of the fundamentals remain the same, typically, there are significant variations between potty training boys and girls.

Knowing the basics of potty training will help your kid become a potty training professional with decreased stress and frustration.

When you start potty education based on gender depends on the individual child when you start potty training. But when you start toilet training, there are several things to remember.

Many girls may be able to start potty training as early as 18 months, or they may not be ready to train potty until they are 4.

When it comes to getting ready for potty training, kids seem to take their time. Boys are usually a couple of months behind girls, and many are not ready until they're at the earliest age of two.

Keep in mind that every child is unique. Your older son could be a potty hero, beginning 18 months of toilet training. Your daughter may not be ready to get started until she is two, and your younger son may not respond until he's three to all this potty talk.

Boys dive on the potty for a few seconds and then stand up and say today's lesson has finished. For certain children, it may be less critical to know how to go to the bathroom if they can go straight into their pants. And we don't think much about wiping people, but we have to remind them to show the penis when they go potty. If you were ever sprayed as a young boy goes into pee-pee, you know why it's necessary.

Looking for the right potty seat is a bit more complicated for boys. Time will quickly be an enormous mess if you're not looking for a potty with a splash shield. This guard stops you from being soaked or bathed when it is time to go peeing or poo. It doesn't matter whether you tell your son to sit while urinating or stand up when it comes to number 2 at the same time, as both will come out at the same time, he still will be sitting, and a splash guard is required.

Although you can find many of the necessary potty time supplies needed to start sharing between genders, certain items vary from girls to boys.

Boys can look like a doll, a doll. It doesn't matter if it's a doll intended to teach kids how to pot or wet a doll. Although they are also reacting to books and DVDs for both sexes, children especially like things that they like, like The Potty Movie for Boys and Potty Superhero.

Moms and dads of boys know that when you're a mom, you have to be on your feet. The same goes for the potty training team. Boys' incentives are bored. A tiny chocolate bar will have to be substituted tomorrow as a reward with a handful of his favorite cereal.

Together with candy, stickers, books, toys, and even the prospect of a trip to the zoo, the movies, or the game store, have a stash of potty training incentives on hand.

The potty training cycle separates boys and girls once more when it comes to discipline and interest. The most important thing to note is to preserve your composure regardless so that your children do not get flooded with feelings that make potty training a traumatic experience.

You've learned girls grow quicker than boys, and that's why you can sit for long periods on the potty with a little girl. She wants to be a broad girl, so she's more polite, so interested in doing the work while she sits on the potty. Most boys believe they have better things to do than they go pee, and their maturity and engagement in potty training are quicker overall. You can also continue to get excited about potty training and then lose interest on the same day.

It is necessary to look for signs of a dissatisfied potty trainer, change the strategies, or even delay potty training.

Girls and boys will have accidents even after they appear to have completed potty training. You'll have to bring with you a change of clothes and wipes a little longer than your daughter's for your son.

Many people don't want to feel dirty. They soon learn that they would have soiled clothing and clothes if they don't interrupt what they are doing to go potty. Accidents happen, but girls avoid them until they know the necessary steps of potty training.

Boys are more likely than girls to have injuries. Some don't mind if they walk around in the back of their pants, with wet clothes or urine. Be prepared for these incidents at home or on the go and ready to change clothes and supplies.

Regardless of gender, don't worry or scold your child if these occur. Making potty training a stressful experience at any point can just allow a few steps back for your kids.

While kids from both sexes can be trained in potty within a few days, a child's average time is around three months. This means that she can understand absolutely when she needs to use the bathroom, goes to the toilet by herself, and requires little to no help in getting washed. Girls typically complete all these potty training steps before boys.

While many boys spend more time in the potty car, they finally cross the finish line. Continue to motivate them and stay optimistic. Your hard work (and yours) will soon pay off.

And what are the specific potty training tips for gender?

Below are several factors that can impact your child's toilet readiness: When teaching your boy, please explain to your kid why he must sit up rather than sit down as a mum or like his sister (if he or she has one). Whenever your child is to go to the potty, put your child right in front of it to try without any trouble.

When your child becomes distracted and starts to move back and forth while peeing, speak to your child about the importance of right-focusing, mainly because of washing and hygiene.

TIP: Try using potty training targets, which are available in several different types. They make peeing a little more fun and motivate your son to produce better results.

Your child needs to learn the correct level of hygiene to prevent harmful germs. Try to remind him that after every bowel movement, it is essential to wash. When he isn't circumcised, he must keep his penis clean by washing under the foreskin.

Your child may not be able to imagine with the potty as a man, that is to say, other than you. It is also easier to involve his father in the entire process. His dad might show him the different body parts required for potty training. Your son would naturally mimic his parent since his biological makeup is identical. Your boys are more likely to learn than girls because girls continue to develop faster–intellectually, physically, and emotionally. You must be more gentle with him because it will take him a little longer to learn the right potty behavior.

When teaching your daughter, tell your daughter that the best way to use the potty is by sitting down. Know how to sit down to avoid leaks.

Proper hygiene. If your child has to clean himself after any bowel movement or even after urination, explain the best way to wash yourself-from front to back to prevent infections of the urinary tract. Also, clarify how necessary it is to wash your hands after each toilet visit.

To speed up the operation, tell her how it is to be done by allowing her to watch you go to the toilet. Observational learning teaches the child the right potty actions more effectively. She also feels more grown-up and more able to learn by emulating you.

The Temperament: Girls of your daughter grow their communication skills faster than boys. Your daughter has a more significant advantage in this regard and therefore saves you more time.

The factors influencing the preparation cycle for boys and girls can be very different. But the main thing is that you still attend to the needs of your kids. While they may have varying physiological needs, the most important thing is continuous care and encouragement and, eventually, the coherence of both sexes.

There are a few more specifics to consider, especially if you have a boy and a girl who need training at the same time. GetPottyTrained.com does a great job of explaining items that must be learned to avoid complications.

When to teach Potty Boys, Do you know the difference between a boy and a girl in potty training?

Learn how to teach potty boys quickly. Education in the toilet boys the variations.

The disparity between potty training for boys and girls is minimal. Boys often take longer than girls to realize what's going on, but the earlier you start to teach your boy, the less obvious that's. It is also easier to potty young boys who sit down instead of standing up, as boys of two and under also find it challenging to focus, target, and pee simultaneously. When your son is a little older and finds it more comfortable to stand and pee, you might want to invent some games that you like. It's a lot of fun to invent a game together and always have a target of some sort to shoot at. You won't have to do this for long, but maybe you want to do this for fun and regular practice once a week.

What to teach potty boys Before boys start training toilets, make sure he is always sent or taken to a bathroom, so he can wait until the very last minute before asking himself whether to use the potty or the toilet. He would have to hurry quickly to the toilet because his bladder is so full that he can not hold on to his pee until he can reach it.

During this early stage of boys ' toilet training, don't ask whether they need to use the bathroom, because almost always they'll say no. It is much easier to tell him when it is time to go to the toilet; he won't hesitate and know that an adult must hesitate "go potty" forward.

Once you start potty train boys first, you need to be very careful. You ought to remember a lot when he used the bathroom last time, what he's doing and how much he had to drink. The better thing for a boy than a girl to train the toilet is that the boys can quickly pee against a tree or even in a quiet spot. Note that you are trying to teach him to learn when to use the toilet. You want to change the behavior and teach him not to do what he's done since he was born. Your child went to the bathroom in his misery for the last year 15- 36 months, and that was OK. The aim now is to break this habit and allow others to use a toilet instead.

Toilet training kids don't have to believe in you and your child and expect to be successful.

Is training potty harder for boys?

The fundamental rule of potty training is preparation. This is true of boys and girls. A kid's slow preparation was long thought to be harder. The truth to this lies in the child's preparation. Very often, boys lag behind girls in their neurological development. Therefore boys might not be as ready as their counterparts for potty training at the same age. Once, it's the child's preparation and not the age.

The common idea is that boys are better taught by adults. Potty Training Boys While this may be the dream, it is not always possible, and the fact is that boys are taught every day by women in the potty. The majority of young boys are best trained by having to sit down first. If there is an issue with your boy who is avoiding the potty when he is sitting on the floor, try putting him back in the toilet.

It might take a little while because he sees others sitting in front of himself, but soon he will adapt, and you will not have as many puddles to clear up. He will sit in front of him until he knows how to channel his stream of urine into the toilet. The remainder of the potty exercise is the same as for boys. Offer him plenty of motivation, praise his accomplishments, and be patient.

Nighttime Potty Training for Boys

It may take a boy a little longer than a girl to do potty training at night. Again, this is related to his slower neurological development. His bladder tells his brain that he has to get up and use the toilet, and he wets his pillow. The use of lightweight sleep pants avoids modifications to night sheets and complaints. It will also help to restrict fluid consumption in the hours before bed.

If your son sees other people using the bathroom, he's going to want to do the same. For safety's sake, it's best left to do so until it's tall enough without a jump. Most boys have mastered it and are comfortable with it when they go to school. In urban legend, a kid's training is a complicated process. With a few changes and with his psychological ability in mind, most parents agree that it was not a nightmare.

SECRETS TO POTTY TRAINING BOYS: HOW TO POTTY TRAIN A BOY FAST

The majority of boys are not potty training boys (unless your son is a peeing prodigy), but they can teach the art quickly and effectively–do not worry, you no longer have to be afraid of sending it to the Pullups under his tuxedo for his first school dance. The main thing is continuity (and incentives–many incentives). Most children go to the toilet if they are allowed to set targets and target high (but not too high–you don't want them to miss the bowl).

This is a long-established (perpetuated) myth that potty boys take longer than girls. One explanation is that women have traditionally learned when little boys might be more open to their daddies.

Another explanation is that girls want hygiene to be better. The average teenage girl is showered with hair and carefully made makeup; the average teenage boy absorbs some body spray and laughs as she flexes in the mirror.

However, for whatever reason, boys can train potty if they want: they just have to learn to go like a kid.

IT'S ALL ABOUT TIMING: Just like the Byrd song says, "To everything, switch. A time for diapers, a time for the potty. "Ok, these aren't the most exact lyrics, but you have a point: it's time for everything. Potty training will never work until your son is ready.

There is no ideal age (though most boys learn to use the potty from 2 to 3 years). Your son must then prove that he is ready to succeed. They may have an interest in the toilet, daily bowel movements, or a dry pair for long periods.

If he shows signs of preparation, it is time to shoot him. Only make sure that you do not start during a transition: for example, when you move into a new home or go on holiday. Then, after you start it if, after an incident, he continues to have, realize that you might have tried too early.

BE Careful IN YOUR Preparation Without a game plan, you wouldn't go into a soccer championship, so you should not fight this war without one. Set the tone first by encouraging him to see an older role model (the Brother or the Father) use the toilet, tell him that everyone is peeing and doing it in the toilet, read books about the subject, encourage him to pick his potty, and make sure that clothing is easily removed. Cute sweatshirts, weak zippers, and buttons.

CULTIVATE COMFORT: People want to be on the toilet by default. This is why they go there with the new New York Times subscription, ready for a long winter crap. Boys are no different: they're not going to do something if anything is awkward. You should, however, cultivate comfort.

Make sure your child rests on the ground with her feet while sitting on the potty (you need a kid-style potty to make this happen).

If you are using a seat adapter, make sure it is comfortable but note that a big the toilet is much scarier than a small one. So make sure your son has a stool so that his feet can be secure.

You're going to want to stop a urine guard as well. You want to shield the floor of your bathroom from the "mansion," but these guards will escape and leave the pot with their pain.

BUY BOY BOY UNDERWEAR AND REWARDS. For kids who can manage their bowels, it is a perfect way of coercion to buy their favorite underwear: they can gladly soil an old pair of short stories, but not one bit of poop can hit Spiderman.

Rewards are also part of the game of potty training. Boys respond particularly to stickers–they like to collect and show them to their friends in binders or jackets. Anything that instills a child's pride motivates them.

SIT DOWN, THEN STAND UP. Allow your son to sit and pee (and poop). Sitting down gives him the chance to learn the basic stuff. When he has mastered it, inspire him to get up, stand up, and pee like the wind (but not in it). But –please be informed–encourage your son to urinate before he's ready for any incidents, and you waste half your food on bleach bottles.

When your son has peeing down, begin target practice.

TARGET PRACTICE. The father best teaches this because he has the right tools. Many parents use adhesives, such as Cheerios or raisins, to make their children want more. At best, your son is irritated by his failure to find a cereal; at least he fishes it out of the bathroom because it is time for a snack. THE Bathroom POOP? YES, IT'S FRIGHTENING. The potty is a normal thing, to Pee, but not Pop. There are a couple of explanations. Your son might be afraid of sitting on the toilet (it's not unusual for children to think that they could slip into the plumbing). Your son could stand and do a poo and don't understand the need to sit. Or your son may face constipation.

Get to the root and work to solve the problem. Don't whine or talk–that's only going to make things worse... like your diaper bill.

MAKE IT SEEM LIKE THEIR IDEA. Kids want to be responsible. Sugar is the only food category if they have their way. A son who is persuaded he was using the toilet is more likely to reuse the toilet (and paint himself in this process as brilliant). Your child is more sensitive if you show your pride.

Prepare MAKES PERFECT-ISH They will prepare to do something positive, like toilet training. Yet training is not enough every so often: consistency is essential. And you must have this continuity.

Make sure that your positivity is consistent–a joke, compliment, inspire. And do not change things: if you start with a child-size potty, continue to use it.

Consider it a precise and fast rule if you have them going to the bathroom before nap time. Do whatever you're doing. It's going to last eventually.

Throughout your journey to John, your pilgrimage to porcelain, there are few helpful tips to guide your trip. Keep in mind: keep naked time aside: naked time is just as it sounds like-let your child run around without clothes. Your son learns to regulate his bladder faster without the protection of a diaper.

Look for clear signals: when you have to use your toilet, most kids display signs–jump or hold onto themselves. Keep an eye out for these hints (and an ear out for a more transparent one (sound of water on the tapestry)).

When your son doesn't take the potty, don't threaten or be disgraceful, as you hoped. This is the quickest way to reverse the cycle.

Take a break if your child doesn't make progress. Then try again within a few weeks–you still have a chance before they are ready. If you somehow don't go to the bathroom after trying and trying again, ask for the assistance of a pediatrician.

KNOW What IS RIGHT ON THE NIGHT: Learning how to regulate your bladder takes much longer than day-long concentration while sleeping. This leaves some children even after they have achieved potty training during waking hours in night slides. Now, there is an indicator that your child can risk the bed without a barrier.

Second, wait until he uses the toilet regularly during the day. After naps and evenings, he starts to test his slide. If it's dry again and again, you can offer a shot at night without diapers. There will still be accidents, so get ready: bedwetting is common among children–about 15% of children aged five and 10% of children aged six still have bed accidents. It can take months or years until your child is free of an accident.

But try it anyway, especially if your child wants to sleep without a paintbox. If nighttime incidents occur, you can always go back to nighttime clothes (but make sure you take them away as soon as he wakes up, or you're going to risk a daytime regression).

By the end of the day (or at the end of the rope), potty training finally occurs. Different children at various times learn proper etiquette. The only thing you can do is go with the flow and wait for the return.

20 HIGHLY EFFECTIVE POTTY TRAINING TIPS

Potty workout tips; Each parent lives with a time devoted to the unpleasant: we say to bowels, let's start this potty! Unfortunately, children will not take to the toilet the way kittens carry their litter for you (and helpful for the detergent industry). But they don't pee in boxes either. So, that's a bonus at least.

Yet, potty training fiercely annoys even the mother and pleased dad–simply put, it's kind of crappy. This is where it helps to learn a few potty tips. It does not guarantee a slide-free life, but it is a strong beginning. Yeah, urine luck when you try:

1. KNOW EACH CHILD IS DIFFERENT: At various levels, every child is on a potty train. Only because the kid potty of your sister learned in 30 seconds (or so she says), you won't have the same experience. The easiest way to teach potty is to have no aspirations first.

2. PRACTICE PATIENCE: Potty training is not easy, and accidents will test everybody's patience. Yet continue to practice serenity. Some kids check you by refusing to use a toilet–don't prove your mistrust works. Keep your temper in check if they piss and pee all over. You don't want them to be scared.

3. Some kids won't use the bathroom for very particular reasons–they may be afraid of something or have had a bad experience. If your child does not want to go, ask them why. The problem could be easy to solve.

4. LET THEM KNOW IT'S NATURAL: IT might be inconvenient to use the toilet, but this is normal. It shows children the underlying need. But don't just show them that everyone has to go, also use your cats. Show them the toilet of your dog (i.e., the backyard) and describe the process. You should also use this opportunity to remind them that yellow snow is not flavored with lemon.

5. Use a timer When you start a potty train, the value of a routine is easy to forget. Diapers didn't need consistency: you changed them when they were dirty. Yet toilet training involves consistently doing the same thing. The use of a timer not only encourages you to allow your child to go but also tells the kid: they hear a chime.

6. Show Happiness AND Discourage: Your children consider you as a superhero when young. We work to change the situation if you are disappointed in them. Use this for your benefit: thank them for using the loo and show disappointment when their underwear is full of poo.

7. REWARDS: There are two good things about childhood: a) your child is happy to pick you up (a soda can or remote), and b) they are reward-driven. The latter is realistic for toilet workouts. There's a lengthy pan of jelly beans or M&Ms. Beware of bribery; however: your child pretends to go to get the products. Therefore, reward when they do something–just pay by drop or plop.

8. MAKE IT FUN: Children like playing; children need to have to play. After all, that's childhood beauty. Kids are more accommodating when you bring this fun to the bathroom. You no longer consider the toilet as less convenient than diapers. Instead, they regard it as useful. So get creative — write a toilet tale that could not stop bursting, sing a toilet paper poem, juggle soap bars at sea.

9. USE A SIZED TOILET: Kids sometimes look at standard toilets as if they are willing monsters to swallow them whole. The use of a children's toilet solves this anxiety, much better if it's cartoon characters. Consider lining the toilet with coffee filters for quick cleanup. Don't use them later to make coffee.

10.   SIT THEM DOWN BACKWARDS: Some children need a toilet with handlebars to sit back. They should grab the lid and hang on to the flight.

11.   Using ART OF AIM, Often, little boys are tougher for potty trains than their female counterparts. Allowing them to aspire for something–a Fruit Loop, a Cheerio, a sad picture of your former flame–motivates them, which they want to be easy to learn.

12.   MAKE THE TOILET: Welcoming Let your children decorate the toilet in whatever way they want. Render it a throne, a palace, a ship with a rocket. Do all you need to do to ensure that the toilet is as accommodating as possible.

13.   COLOR THE WATER: Children like to feel important, and it is essential to be the person who decides the color of the water! Use food or color tablets to transform the bowl to whatever color you want. Hopefully, in no time, the water would be warm.

14.   LIMIT THEIR ACCESS TO TOILET PAPER. About 14 trees die with each child using toilet paper. Simply put, your child uses toilet paper wads and wads if you allow them. Limiting your access saves energy, saves the environment, and prevents you from calling a plumber after each high-fiber meal.

15.   GET THEM AN AUDIENCE: When your child's confidence is not enough to motivate them to go, reassure them. Your neighbor–Hey Henry, come and see what's on our

toilet–doesn't have to ask you to give your child an audience they can talk about: your stuffed toys, your potatoes, or your family dog.

16.   Many children respond better when they see their growth. Monitor PROGRESS A map showing how well they perform motivates them to be moved. Accident-free days: 3.5.

17.   WAKE THEM IN THE MIDDLE OF NIGHT. Even though the child is educated poetry during waking hours, it is more difficult to quash at night. It's one way to stop waking up your child in the middle of the night and pressuring them to go. Tragically, this also ensures that you wake up. So through the just store on overnight diapers instead.

18.   As described above, it is always beneficial to reward your child with gifts. But the surprise factor adds a bit more impact. For one thing, the child's curiosity would not be understood by what they are receiving. On the other hand, their curiosity about the possibilities is also enough to inspire them to go over and over. Who knows, maybe a pony is a surprise.

19.   Giving THEM A Target: Children and adults have specific objectives: to get them out of slides, their target is to be repaid. Compared to a grand finale, this provides a clear target to aim for. You may decide to buy a dollhouse or remote control car for your kid, but only after they are entirely potted. Don't give in first; that's achieving the target.

20.   Learn ABOUT IT All sorts of books on potty training are available. These are all right with you, but they are boring for your babies. Find instead of a children's book on why it is essential to use a toilet. Read it as much as you need with your kids. Let them also read it when they sit on the potty.

HOW TO PREPARE YOUR CHILD AND MAKE TRAINING A LOT EASIER

Potty training is not a sprint, but a marathon. Your kid will finally get there, but the above potty training tips make the process a little easier. They're going to get things moving, at least.

Potty boys can take more time and patience than girls sometimes. Many psychologists and parents believe this is because mothers prefer to do more with children's toilet training than fathers, making it harder for little girls to mimic the process. Regardless of why a boy's potty training can take you longer, so you have to be prepared to be patient.

Tip #1 The first tip is to ensure the readiness of your family.

Watch for signs of preparation, such as that you have a son who wants to use the bathroom or the shower, who wants to mimic older brothers and sisters, who have the signs of independence, who can follow simple directions and respond to positive reinforcement.

Tip #2 Help your son make the potty familiar and relaxed. You need to determine whether an attachment or infant potty seat will be used. If your son is highly interested in either one, go with that option. Many kids may choose to have their potty to help them personalize.

Tip #3 Practice Let your little boy sit on the toilet and get to learn it. If you use a kid potty, you should make it in the space in which he plays and reminds him when it is potty time.

Tip #4 Reward The little boy when he uses the potty effectively. Give him a a special treat or incredible kid right and congratulate him. Tip #5 Make it fun to do a potty workout.

You have to be careful and consistent as a mom. Make your child's reading fun when he is sitting on the toilet. He might also like to watch videos or have a favorite doll or toy stuffed with him.

Tip #6 Using big boy underwear, Do shopping for your son and let him select his favorite underwear. This may be a big reason to no longer wear diapers.

Tip #7 Be careful to Be prepared for crashes and retrogressions. Don't push or blame your boy for incidents. This just contributes to depression and does not encourage your child to use the toilet.

Potty boys are patient and diligent, so it will be worth it when you get rid of the diapers and get your son potty trained for good.

Top 10 Tips For Potty Training Fun

Few people will associate the word "fun" with potty training for babies. But adding a few laughs into this cycle is a perfect way to keep everyone inspired and enthusiastic. Your child should see potty training with some imagination as something to be excited about rather than as a mission.

Books and DVDs-Take the time to include some potty storybooks in your kid's reading time before you continue your training. Give time to talk about the story when you read it if your tot has any questions. Some kids enjoy DVDs, and some excellent DVDs with fun cartoon characters are available to illustrate the toilet training process in clear language.

Sticker map and incentives–Be imaginative as you settle on the incentive scheme to encourage your baby to become confident in the toilet. Tell your child what incentive they want and seek to include this in the process.

Another option is to buy a series of low-cost gifts and wrap them in bright paper (including occasional candy). Small children love to unpack a surprise. Pee-pee song and dance-make a dumb daughter to sing when your kid has a high performance. Make sure it is followed by an equally crazy dance and that you're on a winning mode for fun.

Toilet Goal-Put cheerios or a tennis ball into a toilet for small kids to aim for or add a few drops of blue food to the toilet water so that the wonders of the waters turning to green can be seen by your kid (boy or girl).

Take them shopping for undies-it's very exciting for most children to let your child choose their own "real" undies. This raises enthusiasm and anticipation that when she completes pottery training, she will wear them.

Potty doll or teddy–Use a real doll or teddy and put a little slip so your kids have a friend with whom you can know. As you are a potty trainer for your child, your child will be a teacher for his pet.

Decorate the potty-Let your kid decorate with stickers his potty. She's going to be desperate to use it because she's so proud of it.

Help team–Make sure the family and friends know that potty training is being done. Prepare them so your child can call them and tell them precisely what they've done!

Welcome to the bathroom-Bathrooms are typically very practical (out of necessity). Throw in a few small toys and books to keep your kid occupied during potty seating times. A unique hand towel with its favorite character can make a fun activity with hand drying.

Pleasant food-Constipation is a common issue for children with potty training. Make sure the diet is modified to prevent constipation in foods (including fried food). New foods, such as fresh fruit and vegetables, may be required. Make them more attractive by using either a knife or a cookie cutter to cut into fun shapes.

The most crucial factor to do potty training for children enjoyable is you. Your optimistic, compassionate attitude is crucial to keep everyone focused and productive.

How to teach your young child, are you a mom who wishes to teach your son for the first time? Well, potting is a daunting task, and a boy is typically more difficult to train than a child. That is because it is the mom who trains typically, and it is difficult for a mother to teach her son how a boy should pink. But yeah, don't worry. There are many ways to do excellent potty training for babies.

For a first-time parent, it is essential to remember that potty training should not be a nerve-racking experience for you and your family. While it's a little hard to do, potty training can be done without tension. Below are some tips for proper training:· Buy the materials required two weeks before the first day of potty training.

It is an effective way to train your son for the big day. You can choose to shop with him. Enable him to choose what he wants, from the potty to the pants.

Reveal the potty.

Placing the potty in the playground for your son will encourage him to get used to it. Enable him to do what he wants. Only let him sit on the potty, open it, and put some stuff into it. If he plays on his potty, use it to brace him for his big day. You can use your favorite stuffed animal, for example, to illustrate how it is done. Tell him he'll be a big boy soon and he'll have to do as his stuffed toy does. You may also ask a male relative for assistance in teaching your son how boys are peeing.

Remind your son of his day of training continuously.

Your son should be prepared for the training emotionally. It is, therefore, necessary to speak to him periodically before the actual training day.

Make sure that all resources are available for the actual training.

To order to reduce tension, put the potty, the training pants, and the wipes in an accessible location. Use a timer, too. Make sure your kid goes to the potty every 15 minutes on the first day of school.

Plan for future injuries.

Face it; there will be actual injuries. Bear in mind that your child must not be disciplined. Alternatively, tell him politely he should just pee or poop in the potty.

Thank your child for any accomplishment.

This is important. That is important. Your son will know and be proud of him that he's doing the right thing. You can choose to give him his favorite sweetheart or a fun little toy.

Make training changes appropriate.

It is necessary to track the progress of your child and to change your training strategies based on its response. If the first day of training is successful, the time interval can be modified the next day. For example, on the second day of training, make your son go to the potty every 30 minutes instead of 15 minutes. Continue to adapt until your son is well educated.

In specific ways, this activity can be a little more robust for boys than this activity for girls. But the preparation is undoubtedly successful with the correct implementation of practical techniques. Whether you teach a boy or a girl, it doesn't matter.

Parenting encouragement and preparation of your child

The parent accepts with excitement the achievement of positive potty training. The first moves towards freedom from clothes open up the imagination for the independence that the child one day will accept.

The joy of the parent who knows his role as a saving and independent person is watching his baby develop into a safe and independent person. Yet how to get there best?

Are the same approaches for a boy and a girl?

Do the same methods for boys ' toilets work equally well for girls ' potty training? If you suggest potty training for the 3-year-old, do you ask Aunt Agatha what the best technique your boy could use with her three girls?

If you're a mother with twins, a boy, and a girl, go for the same potty cup. Can you find a different arrangement for each little son and daughter?

Does the Matter of Age?

How can we take this information and extend it to all children with the same brush when we learn the appropriate age for a potty train? How can this knowledge be right for any child, regardless of whether an expert tells you the correct age?

In The Words Of Danny Leviticus, The line from Danny Devito is probably closer to the reality in the great movie "Throw Mamma Off the Train" than the kidding nature of the line implies when it says that "I was trained potty in a pistol." We recognize that the line is intended metaphorically, but even people from the 1940s and '50s can relate to children's nonsense. Self-esteem was a quality that the young boy or small girl might grow anyway.

The parents were there to keep the little tyke independent and confident as soon as possible. Is this an excellent or poor child-rearing method? Were boys and girls who at the age of 18 were outside their doors and themselves in the 1960s better off than the typical kid who wants to use Mom and Dad's welcome mat?

Does Potty Training set the stage for the future?

Toilet training does not predict the future of little Jimmy or Bertha May, but may it set the small tyke down a specific course that would not otherwise be the case?

Some questions should be addressed, if not agonized. Mom and Dad have plenty to think about the crucial role of the next generation's nurturer. But making the right choices on systemic and reasonable questions about childhood can be the difference between a rebellious teenager and a rebellious teenager. Don't underestimate the importance of the potential exclusion of a negative characteristic.

Where to start?

The first step many parents plan to take potty training for girls and toilet training boys into consideration is to learn from the brilliant suggestions other parents will share. Work enables the mother and father to predict problems that may make their essential child-rearing role more satisfying.

Armed with a variety of facts and outcomes as provided by previous speakers, the Parent will predict some of the challenges. Mom and Dad won't be shocked by a strange incident that might be upsetting otherwise.

Through a variety of tales and procedures in your information shop, you can track your child's development and adapt the process to the small child.

And finally, it should be noted that most people undergo potty training, potty training is less important than the relationship between Jimmy or Bertha May and Mom and Dad.

POTTY TRAINING VIDEOS-HOW DO YOU IMPROVE THE PROGRESS OF YOUR CHILD

Potty training videos are beneficial in preparing your child's toilet. There are a lot of people to choose from. These are aimed at inspiring and encouraging children to use the potty.

Many instructional videos also help teach children about their essential body functions. Art and songs are also included. Children have been shown to respond well to music when they learn. It just makes learning more interesting, not to mention. Some videos are animated, while others use actual children to catch the attention of your viewer.

For parents, most potty training videos have additional segments. These segments provide essential tips and guidance to help parents select the right type of potty training for their children.

We all know that kids mimic what they see. This is why it is so critical that parents keep a watch on television and in films for their children. If you ask them to go potty, it's no different. They may want to emulate what they do in videos as it allows them to become a big boy or girl. You can always be confident it feels more comfortable to be clean and dry than on a wet or messy diaper. Some videos also have the right toilet skills to use the potty for them.

Many toilet training videos, including "Once Upon a Potty" (for him or her), are around for a long time. That's a classic. Several parents and kids watched this video together to make the training successful. This video is useful for parents who want to ski through potty training seats and learn to use a big toilet right away. This idea does not work for all children, but the video teaches children not to be afraid of the toilet. "Go Potty Go" is another lovely potty training video. This video is described as small children. This is to help them understand what they need to do to go alone to the potty. The silly songs, stories, and games are designed to inspire your child to use the potty successfully interactively.

Are you a mother who would like to train your son for the first time? Okay, potty exercises are demanding, and the training of a boy is typically more complicated than that of a girl. It's because it's the mother who trains typically, and it's tough for a mother to teach her son how a child should pink. But yeah, don't worry. There are different ways to teach potty boys effectively.

For the first time, your parents will note that potty training should not be a the stressful task for you and your family. While it is a little challenging to do, potty training can be practical without stress. Here are some tips that can help you complete a training course: · Purchase the necessary materials two weeks before the first day.

It is an effective way to train your son for the big day. You can choose to shop with him. Enable him to pick what he wants, from the potty to the shoes.

Reveal the potty.

Placing the potty in the play area of your son will encourage him to get used to it. Enable him to do what he wants. Let him sit down on the potty, open it, put a few items into it. If he plays on his potty, use it to brace him for his big day. For example, your favorite stuffed toy can be used to illustrate how it is done. Tell him he'll be a big kid soon, and he will do what his stuffed toy does. You may also want to ask a male relative for guidance to teach your son how boys are peeing.

Remind your son regularly about his training day.

Your son should be prepared for the training emotionally. It is also essential to speak to him about it periodically before the actual training day.

Make sure all supplies are available for the actual preparation.

In an accessible location, position the potty, training pants, and wipes to avoid stress. Using a timer, too. Try to get your kid to the potty every 15 minutes on the first day of school.

Plan for future injuries.

Face it; things are going to happen. Keep in mind that your child will not be disciplined. Tell him then politely that he should just pee or poop in the potty. Reward your child for any achievement.

This is important to do. Your son has to learn and believe he does the right thing, and you are proud of him. You can choose to play him with his favorite sweetheart or a fun little ball. Make training changes appropriate.

It is necessary to track the progress of your child and change your training strategies based on its response. If the first day of training is good, the time interval can be modified the next day. For example, on the second training day, make your son go to the potty every 30 minutes rather than 15 minutes. Continue to adapt until your son is well educated.

This activity for boys can, in some ways, be a little harder than for girls. Nevertheless, the preparation can undoubtedly be efficient with the correct implementation of practical techniques. Also if you train a boy or a girl, it won't matter.

Potty Training Tips – How to incorporate the small ship, you must first select which ship to use.

Your children can use an adult toilet, a smaller toilet seat, or their bowl. When you make a purchase, bring your child and let her engage in the process. Enable them to pick their potty or toilet and make sure they make a superior choice.

When you go home, let your young man open the package and find the item you bought and help them mount it in the bathroom. If you want her to use the bathroom, you need a step stool. Perhaps you want your child to help you pick this.

Take the time to visit your favorite child's shop's big boy or girl underwear department. When you let your youngster choose his undies, you will tell in an excited voice that he will still be able to display his new underwear.

Your main goal is to excite your child about the potty training to come. Once you have agreed on the new seating arrangements together with your kids, Let your child get used to just sitting with or without the diaper.

You'll want to provide your child with some entertaining entertainment.

Many popular entertainment options include comics, color cards, pencils, musical instruments, or other portable toys.

Allow the bathroom with a beautiful place to visit. When your child likes music, you can take her favorite tunes on the radio and play them.

You don't want your child to be depressed, so don't just start making incentive maps.

You are just adding the potty first, so just keep it relaxed and try to make it fun.

In the last few days before the training: use supportive and constructive words to let your child know what is going on.

Choose a day you expect to continue and remember the whole week ahead. Your child will know what to expect and will be able to respond with signals that she is ready. When she says, "no," don't give up hope when you tell her what's coming.

Maybe she will be ready when the day arrives finally, but don't be surprised if she shows fear.

Let her think it's all right if she's not ready now, and in a few days, she can try again. You may be shocked if he wants to do it all by himself.

If there are issues, I'd recommend that you stop taking a couple of days about potty training and then start a new day again.

A perfect idea for training Potty Makes sure both mother and father and all children are aboard. All caregivers must follow the approach you have chosen for potty training. Make sure that someone who can help you learn the technique and what you expect from it.

There are all sorts of potty training videos, as you can see. There are just a handful of highlights. It's a smart idea to use a video to inspire your little one to use the potty. It could simplify the whole process for you both.

LAZY MOM'S POTTY TRAINING FOR TODDLERS

My kids taught potty. It was quick.

Until I clarify, here is a history where kids come from current ideas about toilet training.

During the 1940s, Dr. Benjamin Spock (no, not Mr. Spock) wrote "Baby & Child Care." He suggested plans to take the infant to the bathroom on all occasions before the infant had an accident at the potty. The parent recompensed the child with candy or a cheap toy, and eventually stopped practicing. The beginning of Spock was when the baby was a year and a half. That is how my mother taught me. Many people used Spock in the 1970s.

Additional advice was to wait until the child was fully mature when the child started offering his toys to people. So said the experts.

The reward principle was time-tested. Another suggestion was to have a child's potty chair in the bathroom by the time the children were around a year old.

Rather than clothing and paper diapers, no disposable pull-ups or wetting tools were available at night. There were just extra tight training pants and standard pants of cartoons and superheroes. That was the target.

In 1977, I gave birth to my son. I put the potty chair in the bathroom when he was one year old, and he saw his parents use our big one. He was often sitting on him, lid up, lid down, on his diapers, just a second just two before his bath without a break.

When he was two, I started teaching him seriously, potty. The scheme of incentives almost destroyed the bank. I rewarded him for two weeks with tiny plastic creatures, dinosaurs, and sometimes M&M, all of which become more expensive each day. Instead, I decided to cut back slowly. My son didn't get his goody for the first time, he reverted. No reward, no actions. I knew he knew what he was going to do. He was too smart.

I tried the same dumb tactic again to justify my lack of brains. We found thickly lined Big Boy pants on a shopping expedition. I bought a pair. At home I showed my son the shoes, I asked him what they were for, and I said that he had to come and let me know when he was ready to be a big boy.

Then I put them in the fridge.

He came to me one day and told me that he needed his pants for Big Boy. I gave them to him. Following that, he had an incident in bowel movement. I took him to the garden, telling him that I had to clean his big boy pants myself from then on. It was his only accident.

When he educated himself, he was three years old.

Seven years later, I gave birth to a daughter. I did not want to do bonuses. I learned that children want to behave like adults and want to be trained. The little potty was in the bathroom from the time she was a year old. We purchased some Big Girl pants when she was about 1 1/2. The big lined ones she didn't like. She wanted the characters of cartoons. I got them and put them in the fridge waiting for the day she was ready to be a Big Girl. She said she needed them one day.

She had just one mistake, and we went to the garden spigot in the backyard. She got her pants washed, and that was her only mistake. She was one and a half.

"What did you do?" my mother's age teacher asked, our Mother's Day Out. "Nothing," I said with a smile.

There is a lot of information about training in toilets, self-help books, products, online videos, books bought from the store, or nothing you can do. Potty kindergarten teaching is rarely easy work. What most parents do is use diapers at night for most children who undergo potty training. It gives your child a bit of protection at night and helps them to concentrate during the night on the most important thing.

It's okay if you look for signs that indicate your kid knows what they're doing, like when they're wet or when they think it's time to go to the loo. It's a sign they're set.

As a parent, you must know that potty training for girls is a separate undertaking for men. Nine out of ten in a family situation, the potty teacher, is usually a female, and little girls find it easier to learn from someone they can model. If you have an older brother or your little boys 'dad in the house, invite him to go to the toilet with him so he can know by modeling.

Many parents find it fun and pleasant to use incentives and rewards during potty training to improve the child's actions. Another perfect way to improve your little girl or boy's proper potty training is to use a variety of videos.

You can pick them up in a nearby department supermarket, a supermarket like Mothercare, or even a bookshop. The books will probably be fun. Such books, which can be put in cards, demonstrate the entire process of using the potty and executing the operation. It is also best to encourage your child to look at them when they are potty.

Potty Training Tips-Simple Ways to Train Your Toddler

Start Early: it doesn't mean your kid can sit on the pot, and success is right here. It just means that you will launch the concept early. At 14 months, begin to talk about the potty and read potty books. I know that some parents don't think they should use the word 'potty' and only use the word 'toilet' because later it will be confusing. That's simply not valid. When they are 2 or 3 years old, they know the difference, and when they're younger, I wouldn't think about that. I think kids enjoy the thought of getting a potty of their own. Only make it unique for them by thinking about what a good kid they are and what else will happen.

Pull-ups are not needed: Yes, they are friendly and often handy, but I think it's better just to put on underwear. Select times or on a weekend where you can have some severe potty workouts and just enjoy some fun undies (such as Diego or Dora). They'll be so excited because they're wearing their big boy!

You want to make sure you don't stain your exclusive underwear. I think that pull-ups make it too easy to bring them in. You want it to be awkward because if you pee in your undies, that's going to be. When you're out of your room, you might still use pull-ups, but I think at home, you are undied, or nothing is better. At first, there is no time between "mommy, pee-pee" and an accident.

Prizes: Oh yeah, ensure that you've got plenty of them. "I'm going to give you a bonus if you go to a potty of pee." That is your famous line. This can range from stickers to sweets. Warning: if you use sweets, then good luck, try again to offer some other prizes! One tactic for incentives is to claim that if you go pee and two stickers if you go poop, you get a sticker. Try to make it fun, or you'll feel obliged, and it'll make it harder for you! Make sure that you follow through, like everything else. They don't get a bonus if they don't go potty.

The Method: I think the way you do potty workouts depends on your kids. For others, it's going to work in a potty boot training camp, where you can practice for three days straight. They will wear just a painting to bed during this period. When awake, don't pinch and brace for many incidents! For some, just be careful and let your child know when they're ready. Often a baby needs to go into the potty and feel like a big boy, so it might be appropriate to get him. Finally, just relax – it's not like your little one would be 10 (I hope not at least), and wear a slip!!

Outside the house: make sure it's ready! Bring a potty with you if you are driving an SUV or minivan. It can be faster and more convenient for you than finding a toilet. Have a spare dress change in your car, and always remind you're a child if they need to go potty. Look for signs like pee-pee dance. When an accident happens, just try to relax because you don't want to embarrass your kids.

Nighttime: Potty training can be most challenging at bedtime. Nighttime: You can wonder, how can your child go all night long? Only leave this part to think about at the very last point. Focus on during the day and wear a pull-up or a diaper during the night. Upon finally getting ready for this point, make sure a potty is near the bed. Have a new sheet and pajamas in the area, if only you wake up from the bunk. When that isn't first, they may also not be able to hold their pee through the night. Be patient, and your child will soon be ultimately potty trained.

Boys: The best tip for a child is that when you start potty training, it's to sit for peeing. Make sure your peepee is pointing! You do not want to overwhelm him with much detail; he has enough to think about it. You should incorporate the idea of getting up to go pee as time goes by. The best thing to do is to see Papa in the shower. What?! What?! Sure, it's essential. We are leading by example, and now he can be like papa. It's going to work! When you follow the advice above and try not to stress yourself out about potty training, it will just happen. Seek to be fair and note that toddlers are smart and, at this age, want to feel like a big boy. Make it unique, and before you know it, you will have a toddler who is potty trained.

POTTY TRAINING FOR GIRLS IN THREE DAYS

A COMPREHENSIVE GUIDE ON HOW TO HELP YOUR DAUGHTER QUICKLY AND FASTER

SUCCESSFUL POTTY TRAINING FOR GIRLS

Many parents are facing a difficult situation in terms of training their kids; the most common problem is the time to begin potty training. People assume potty training is better for girls than doing the same thing with boys, but there are things to consider before making assumptions. The most important thing is that the boys must learn two toilet tricks, one by sitting down and the other by using the toilet while standing. The girls must learn only one way that takes probably less time. It is a time-consuming job to teach your girl to use the toilet properly, and you need to be very sure that your child is ready for this work before you start the process. If the time isn't right, and you want to move your child for preparation, the phase will undoubtedly take off, and it takes longer than your wishes or hopes.

The children, regardless of whether they're boys or girls, learn to mimic their parents or other family members, so it's essential for you to be a mother and to be your girl's role model. Potty girls are easier to teach, and if you let them watch the toilet and other stuff in the bathroom, she will continue to mimic you and continue to do precisely the same. If you see any signs from your girl of these imitations, you can be sure that it's time for the training to start and make it comfortable in the toilet. Different research indicates that the ages of 18-20 months are considered to be the ideal start to potty training, although, for this, there are no hard and fast guidelines. The first thing to teach your child is to use the toilet and let them use the toilet safely if they feel the need to pull or potty. You should get your girl a pot and allow her to sit on the seat with or without nappies often during the day, then move on to the next step of sitting on the bench, without any nappies or underwear.

Besides encouraging the child to use the toy-power seat, it is also necessary to note any apparent indications that your child is having bowel movements or wishes to pink. Whenever you look, take your girl to the toilet and make her sit on the toilet. Potty training girls can be tiring and sometimes the unintentional mess can be cleaned but do not punish or reprimand your girl, which makes them apprehensive of the training, but instead encourages them to tell you and visit the toilet. Once you feel that the movement of your girl's bladder and bowel is correctly controlled during the day, you will start your toilet and potty night training.

Potty looks like a replica of a toilet bowl compared to a real toiled bowl. You'll miss several things once your baby grows up. It doesn't pay to be hurried: it takes you time and patience and a reasonable degree of cooperation and encouragement to teach your daughter how to use the potty.

Potty training isn't something that people love: nobody seems to enjoy long beach walks, golf, and E-coli exposure. But, if you're a dad, the land comes with it. Hold strong–your daughter is going to follow suit.

To most parents, it is difficult to know when to start potty training for a child. When to start potty training-the best potty training age; of course, your child sometimes asks you. You tell them tales of the big prizes, which emerge after they use the bathroom, and they're immediately able to pee and punch.

And how do you know when a child is ready? You will look for signals, both visible and subtler (actual signs that read "Must Tinkle in Toys Toilet").

So let's take a moment before we get there to make sure you're comfortable first. There's some sensitivity you need in the bowels fight. You should also be aware of this fact:

KNOWING YOUR STATISTICS. You might have changed many pitchers to a science! Don't worry–you're not the only parent you've got. Parents are potty, older, and older babies. In the United States, not only has the average age increased, but it has also increased in Brazil, China, and Switzerland.

Now children are being raised in the potty for an average of three years rather than a few months in two years. The universal availability and usability of the units are one explanation for this.

KNOWING THE RIGHT POTTY TRAINING AGE. You have to know when you and your child are going on potty trains. Studies show that preparation is optimal between 27 months and 32 months. Start too early and start too late makes your child more vulnerable to bed weeping and injuries. However, every child is different: it probably won't work for one of your kids. It'd be too fast.

Good luck to you, experts suggest potty girls learn early, and girls aren't upset so quickly. Children with older siblings who look up and mimic the toilet train can also be more straightforward.

The secret to proper training is only beginning if your daughter is ready to do so. While some children may begin as early as 18 months, others may not be able to learn until they are three or four.

Girls Potty training Successful training depends on starting when you're sure your daughter is ready. Your daughter may be willing to start potty training as early as 18 months or not ready until she is four. Most parents start between 2 and 3 years.

Girls are usually trained about three months earlier than boys, but it's not a complicated and fast rule. If she has older siblings, she will know before she was born.

Choose your time attentively. It is best to avoid beginning training when significant changes occur, including starting at the kindergarten or the arrival of a new sibling. She could feel overwhelmed to face a new challenge.

Waiting until she is finished will help to get potty training right at the beginning.

If your child starts to say "no" to everything, please remember that it is only a phase. She'll pass it, but perhaps you want to postpone potty training until it's over.

Studies show that when parents initiate potty drills before a child can be physically or emotionally willing, it just takes longer. In other words, once you start, you arrive at your destination simultaneously. First, use this checklist to see if your daughter is ready for potty training.

POTTY TRAINING PREPARATION CHECKLIST

You still wanted to adjust the first slide yesterday, and now you wonder if it is time to start potty training. Children are not magical until they are ready to learn how to use potty, but some acquire the physical and cognitive skills required between the ages of 18 and 24 months.

Many parents do not start potty training until 2 1/2 to 3 years old when their baby's healthy bladder controls are trusted. And some kids don't want to practice potty until they're up to three, or even four.

The quality of training depends more on the maturity of your kid than on the age.

Focus on timing until you have decided that your daughter is ready. Be sure your child's routine is well defined–it might not be more open to change if she has just begun preschool or a new sibling or felt ready to face up to a new challenge.

Use the checklist below to test the progress of your baby towards readiness and keep in mind that starting before your child is ready does not mean you will end sooner.

Avoid times where her usual aversion to infants is strong and wait for new thoughts to become available. To teach, follow the steps:

Let her watch and learn to imitate, and it is a simple first step to watch you use the bathroom. It is essential to be specific when thinking about body parts. When you tell her to call her "wee-wee," her vaginal part, because each other's name sounds more formal, she can assume that her genitalia is humiliating.

If your daughter sees her older brother, dad, or a preschool or daycare friend standing high in your bathroom, she'll most likely want to try and stand up. Have her. Let her. Sure, a couple of messes have to be cleaned up, but hopefully, very soon, she will understand that she has no equipment to make things work, so you won't have to involve her in a power fight.

If she continues, look at you and explain how moms and their daughters will sit down to pink.

Buy the right equipment: Many experts advise you to buy a child-size pot that your kids will believe is their own and which is more comfortable than a full toilet. (Many kids are afraid to fall into the toilet, and their fear can hinder potty training.) The toilets may be a dangerous place for curious kids, so always supervise them when they use the toilet.

Whether you prefer to buy a toilet adapter, make sure it feels comfortable and secure and fits tightly. If you go along this path, you're going to have to stool your daughter, because it's crucial that she can easily navigate the toilet any time she needs to go. She must also be able to stabilize herself on her feet if she has a bowel movement.

You may want to pick up some photo books or videos for your daughter that make it easier for her to get all this new information. Fill out, Oh, yeah! Find out, Uh! Have to Go! Or Once Upon a Potty, which also comes with a doll and miniature potty edition.

Help your child get clean with the potty. This child needs to get used to the idea of using the potty early in the process. Start by letting her know that her very own potty chair. You can customize it by writing your name or having it decorate with stickers. Then try to lie on it with her shoes.

For a week or two, you might recommend that she try it down with her shoes. If she seems resistant at all, stop the temptation of pushing her. It will only create a power struggle that can ruin the entire cycle.

Remember to use it for potty lessons when your kid has a favorite doll or stuffed toy. Many kids love seeing their favorite toy turn and should learn more about this than asking them what to do. Some parents also create dolls or stuffed animal toilets. And her favorite doll will sit on her potty while the child's chair is perched.

Keep your daughter focused on the benefits of potty training by taking her on a particular order: Buy panties. Let her realize that she can do whatever she wants. (Underwear with a favorite movie character or colorful logo is usually a big hit.) Talk up the excursion in advance, because she's excited to be old enough to wear potty and underwear just like a mom or her big sister.

Build a training schedule: To get your child out of the slides depends on your routine and whether your daughter is in daycare or preschool. If it is, you would want your plan to be coordinated with your kindergarten provider or instructor.

You will determine whether to use the back-and-forth system for moving from slides to jackets or the Cold Turkish system for full-time underwear. Some experts suggest changing into plastic pants that are practically like clothing but can be pulled up and down like underwear.

But some argue the switching to underwear and old cotton shoes is preferable, which will help your daughter know like she's wet instantly. That, of course, makes it more likely that any incidents will be cleaned up.

You will have to decide for yourself and your child what is best. The doctor of your child can recommend one way or the other.

You'll want to start using diapers at night for at least a while. And your daycare provider or preschool teacher should worry about when to go to classes.

Know her to sit down and clean. One of the main things your daughter needs to know is how to clean correctly. Explain that she has to make sure she transfers the bowel paper from the front to the back to prevent infection. When it is too hard for her to understand (and it can happen to many girls because it needs to know that she has to go some way), teach her to dry up the area after she has peed.

Although rare, bladder infections tend to be more common in girls at the time of potty training. If your daughter must urinate regularly or thinks she has to go unexpectedly, she claims she is uncomfortable or complaining of stomach pain, or begins to pee her pants after proper bladder management has been set up, call her doctor to get it tested.

Set aside some time naked. Nothing makes your kid find out whether she wants to go for some time without a diaper. Place the potty in an open area and allow her to sit frequently on it.

Look for signals (springing up and down, keeping her legs together, or swaying side by side), use these signals to indicate that it is time to do well.

You can do this for several days in a row, in the evenings while the family is together or on weekends. The more time the child spends on slides, the more it learns.

Celebrate victories. She will have a few spills, but hopefully, your daughter will realize how much she can get in the pot. Celebrate with fanfare this moment. Reinforce the belief that she has achieved a considerable achievement by giving her a "big girl" right, for example, to have an extended bedtime.

Try not to make a lot of the journey to the potty, or your child will start to feel anxious and alert under the light of all this scrutiny.

When she doesn't excel at first, try again. The more she uses her potty, the better she'll be at it. But you should do some things to make it easier for her. Dress your child in casual clothes that she can take away easily or buy sweets too large.

Don't overreact or punish if she still has trouble with the idea. Nothing will ruin potty training more quickly than making a child feel guilty about an incident. Typical injuries are part of the operation.

Be mindful that even children who regularly use the bathroom for months still encounter incidents when they are participating in an operation. If you are irritated, note that scolding her for wetting her pants means months ahead. So if you're still upset, take a break for a couple of weeks and then try it again.

Raise the fun factor. Your child will more likely remain motivated during the entire process if you approach potty training with a little panache. Drag a little blue food into the bathroom, and she will be shocked by how she can turn the watercolor. Place her favorite book next to the toilet in the magazine rack so she can see it whenever it is needed.

You may suggest providing incentives if your child begins to lose interest when she is well into potty training. One common way to chart her accomplishments is to use stickers and a calendar.

Whenever she goes to the potty, she may add a sticker of her choice to the tab. Looking at the riches of the sticker will keep her motivated.

If the stickers are not enough, you can provide a new incentive, such as a trip to the park or a gift you like, when they collect enough sticks or stay dry for several days in a row. For potty training suggestions.

Shift into Night Mode You can step into the next process after your daughter has a hold of day-long preparation. Wait until she is healthy and potty, then start to check her diapers in the morning and nap to see if they are dry. In the day, several children can stay dry after about six months after learning to use the toilet.

She is still under training at night is more complicated since it depends on the body's ability to retain the urine for an extended period and how deep it sleeps. If she decides to try sleeping, go ahead and let her go. A soft mattress cover will help if you are worried about her soiling the mattress.

If she isn't able to stay dry after a couple of nights of the experiment, put it in a non-judgmental way. Tell her that her body can not do the next step and assure her that she'll be strong enough to try again soon.

If your child is dry for three of five nights, make your policy "all pants, all the time" official. Encourage her attempts to stay dry by restricting how much she drinks after 5 p.m. And get her up before you go to bed for a bathroom ride.

Ditch the slides. Once your child can say farewell to the slides, she's accomplished a lot. Realize this and improve her pride in her accomplishment by letting her give her remaining diapers to a family of younger children, or by packing up her tissue slides and giving them the last time via the painting service. Or encourage her to choreograph a jig around the house and name it "no more slides." When nature calls, the whole family will form a conga-line and go to the potty.

SIGNS YOUR KID'S READY TO GO POTTY

Children can not control their bladder or bowel movements before the age of 12 months, and some children who display several signs of preparation are still unable to control their removal physically. But kids who can stay dry overnight can take longer to stay dry overnight. Indeed, you may want to think of day and night dryness as two different milestones for potty training. You don't have to wait for every element to start training, only look for an independence pattern and an understanding of what it means to be in the bathroom like an adult. To help you get started, read the positive potty training techniques.

The effectiveness of potty training depends more on preparation than on your child's age.

Visual signals are often synchronized to walk and even to run.

She urinates at one time a decent volume and has frequent, well-formed bowel movements at predictable intervals.

She has "dry" intervals of 2 hours or more or during naps, indicating that her bladder muscles are adequately formed to retain urine.

Behavioral symptoms

Can sit quietly for 2-5 minutes in one spot.

Could pull up and down his pants.

Dislikes a wet or dirty diaper feeling.

Shows a curiosity in the behaviors of others (would like to watch or wear underwear to go to the bathroom).

Give a physical or verbal indication if she has a bowel movement like grunting, squattering, or asking you.

It indicates a desire for freedom.

She takes pride in his achievements.

It's not difficult to learn to use the bathroom.

It is not harmful or contrary at a generally cooperative level.

Cognitive signs

Recognize the physical signals, which means that she needs to go and warn you before it happens, or even hold it until he has time for the potty.

Can obey basic directions, like "go get the toy."

Understand how important it is to place items where they belong.

Has urine and stool names.

10 Indicators OF POTTY READINESS

Until your kid is ready to start, other indicators of readiness for potty training, include:

1. THEY HAVE Less WET DIAPERS: If your kid's painting has been planned regularly and is only ready every few hours to turn to the toilet. This is a sign that they begin to regulate, which is vital for the regulation of the bladder.

2. THEIR BOWEL MOVEMENTS ARE PREDICTABLE. A kid who pulls in time off the potty before anything happens. If you know that your child is always about 8 a.m., you know you're ready with the toilet. It raises the probability of proper potty training.

3. THEY ARE THEIR Bodyshop. How do you think you have to go? How do you feel you have to go? Your body tells you! Your body tells you! Children who can listen to their bodies are better suited for the potty than children whose desires and distress are ignored. A child with a body sensitivity will grunt, squat, or cover from pseudo-privacy under a table.

4. The use of the toilet requires more flexibility than the use of a diaper. Children must, first of all, be able to remove their clothing. They're potty prepared if your kid can do this.

5. THEY UNDERSTAND DIRECTIONS. Most kids think they don't know what's going on. It never really changes for children-adolescents too! But it's time for your kid to take the diapers if it can follow clear instructions –stuff like "go potty" and "sit down."

6. THEY Will SIT FOR SEVERAL MINUTES Make sure they will stay quiet before putting your child in the toilet. You don't want your child to use the pot when they get up and open the midpoop door.

7. When your child runs around the house, singing, "I'm always baby here, I roar!"They want freedom, you know. Girls who want to establish themselves as heads of households are more likely than girls to attend toilet training.

8. THEY COMPLAIN ABOUT BEING WET. They're ready for underwear if you have one kid who doesn't like wet in a wall.

9. THEY'RE CURIOUS ABOUT THE BATHROOM. If the child asks questions about the bathroom–where toilet paper goes when they're flushed, why do people go, be it moms or daddy picks and dumbbells? Girls tend to be like their parents, and they'll want to be like that when they see you out of diapers (hopefully you are!).

10.   THEY TELL YOU THEY Want TO GO. Maybe the sure sign that your little girl is ready to use the toilet is most natural. When children learn how to communicate their wishes, let them loose, and fulfill their porcelain dreams.

HOW DO YOU ENSURE A SMOOTH PROCESS

Now that you know how to say if the timing is right, how do you ensure a smooth process? That's a severe problem–a smooth operation you can't guarantee! There's something likely to go wrong. But the following doses and can not help control damage.

SO, DO: Let your child run naked: it makes your child become more at peace with its body and what it's trying to mean. Without a diaper, it is impossible to avoid pee!

Stop clothes with buttons: you think it's challenging to use clips, buttons, and zippers? Attempt to be three!

Pay attention: kids who are practicing potty don't suggest that they have to go five minutes in advance: their window is more like ten seconds. Pay attention; therefore –if you don't, your child can eventually water the fern in the living room.

Lobby offer: all hail the poo! The more you do, the more your child will be proud of you.

Motivation: One of the best ways to inspire your kid is to remind them that they're growing up with the toilet as a big boy.

"Toilet, Tammy, add the potty. Tammy, shower! Shower!" The exposure to your child's potty makes it less scary. Do bring it up as soon as you can. Let your child see you use the bathroom, take your dolls or toys, and read books. Do what you can to make your child happy –comfort is crucial.

Practice proper hygiene: the best way to provide your child with good hygiene is from the beginning. Make sure your child is always brushing, flushing, and washing his hands with soap and water. Do you run your hands under a halving second? It just doesn't count. Seek to wash for a long time, about half a minute.

Check for dryness: When your child's diaper stays dry, show them that you're proud. However, don't blame or threaten if the diaper is damp–this can lead to regression.

SPEAKING OF DON'TS, Always REFRAIN FROM:

Expecting miracles: A kid who takes to the toilet like a duck takes to water isn't reality. Expecting too much just sets the stage for disappointment.

Punishing: As described above, any punishment will lead your child to backslide. Never punish for pee or poop–just dissuade them from future endeavors.

Food or drink is retained: Many parents use liquids (or things like bran) to teach potty. But you should do the opposite–bring on the juices! The more they have to go, the more practice they get.

Use the force: Potty training should never be pressured–this will lead to frustration and make your child more resistant the next time around.

Fighting a losing battle: Not every kid potty trains on the first attempt (or the first twenty attempts). When you 're losing the fight, accept defeat. Seek again in a couple of weeks.

Losing your willpower: But to try again does not mean that you never try. You will finally teach your child potty. When you don't, until the mid-fifties, they will live in your cellar. When you still don't go to the bathroom after trying and trying again, get a pediatrician's support.

Note, timing is vital when it comes to the potty! Never begin this journey during periods of stress or change (such as going on vacation or the birth of a new sibling). And don't let anger get your best: you can prove victorious in bowels war, but it takes time.

Potty training is a parental power test, but persistence is nothing, and Clorox can't remedy it. The best way to ensure a smooth transition from the paint to the pot and not again is to make sure that your kid is ready to sit on his throne and reign over the land of laminate tiles.

FREQUENTLY ASKED QUESTIONS ON POTTY TRAINING

WHAT DO I NEED FOR POTTY TRAINING?

Start by buying a pot and tell her it's her potty. You could let her personalize it with genius stickers or write on it her name. Your daughter can feel safer with a pot than with a full-size toilet.

Some kids are reluctant to fall into the toilet, and sometimes potty training will interfere. A potty is comfortable to sit on, get on and off, and walk around the house comfortably.

When your daughter can learn to use the bathroom together, make it as quick as you can. You should try an exercise seat that sits on top of your toilet. It must feel relaxed and safe and bind firmly, without wobbling. You will also need to take a measure to help her get on and off the seat.

Reading image books, using a potty training app, or seeing a potty training video can make it more enjoyable for her.

How will we begin training potty?

Children learn by imitation. With an open bath policy at home, your daughter has plenty of chances to see how you wee.

She may remember you are sitting down, and Papa is standing up to the toilet. This is your chance to give the mechanics a brief guide on how boys and girls use a toilet.

To make your child acquainted with the concept of using the potty, begin by suggesting that she sits with her nappy on the potty. You should demonstrate how to sit there with your favorite doll or stuffed toy.

Don't push her if she's resistant to it. You can just build a power war that could disrupt the whole cycle.

How can I get her to use the potty?

Spark the curiosity of your daughter is potty training for her to pick her knickers on a special shopping trip. Favorite cartoons are typically a big success.

Speak up about the trip in advance. She would be pleased that she is old enough to wear potty panties, just like her big sister or Mummy.

When are we ready to banish nappies?

Consistency is essential to get your kid out of clothes. Whether you are in a kindergarten with a child, child, or family, make sure everybody has the same approach.

Ideally, you can go straight to full-time underwear to avoid confusion for your boy. Sweeping is a choice, but your daughter feels more instinctively when she's soaked with real pants or washable cloth training pants. Be prepared for the occasional accident along the way, whatever you use.

It is a good idea to pack your daughter with a clean pair of cuddles, buckles, and pants while you're out, even if you only hit the shops. At least for some time, you'll want to go on long trips with nappies or disposable pants at night. If you can't decide what to do for the better, see if other parents in our support group have ideas or speak to mothers. Your health visitor is also a valuable source of assistance and guidance.

Treat your daughter to wipe from front to back, particularly when she has a poo, to avoid transmitting bacteria from the bowel into her vagina and urethra when it's too difficult for her to clean from front to back, simply teach her how to pull dry after she wees and call you when poo is over.

Infections of the urinary tract are not widespread in infants but are more prevalent in girls than in boys. Take her to the doctor when she has to: pee more often or has a sudden urge to go claims that it hurts to pee and complains of tummy or pelvic pain wet her pants after a strong bladder control.

Let her be without clothes for a moment. Place the potty anywhere she can quickly reach while she plays and allows her to sit there over and over again. Be ready for the occasional puddle–have the tapestry cleaner available, or seek to place plastic over the tapestry.

Keep an eye out for signs that she has to go from foot to foot, grin, and place her hands between her thighs. Then say it's time for potty. Do it for several days, at night, or even at weekends. The more time she spends out of her shoes, the quicker she knows.

Where will I compliment her when studying pottery?

Your daughter eventually gets it into the pot after a few painful mistakes. Celebrate this vital achievement by watching her favorite cartoon or reading a new bedtime story. Don't go crazy and do a lot of any potty ride. Too much attention will make your child feel anxious and self-aware.

Why will I treat potty accidents?

Keep trying. The more she does it, the better she will be at it, as any talent your child masters do. See what you can do to improve things for her. Dress her up in casual clothes that she can take off quickly. Tell her to use this potty instead of asking her (the normal response is "no"), and allow her to read a book later. Don't make her feel guilty if she has an accident. Even kids who have used the bathroom for months suffer accidents.

It can be irritating, but it can mean more months of nappies than less to tell her to wet her pants.

How can I have fun teaching potty?

If your daughter gets lost in potty training, offer to pay for it.

Whenever she wees or does a pot in her pot or asks you to go, she can add a sticker to the wallboard or fire up her potting app. Once the reward stickers are put, they inspire her to continue to try. When she has ample wallcharts or device incentives or stays dry for a certain amount of days, it is time for a treat, like a long-awaited toy.

When are nights going to be dry?

When your daughter is educated in the potty, check at her nappies in the morning and after naps to see if they are dry. If she's dry a few nights in a row, it's time for a nighttime game plan.

Some four-year-olds aren't dry at night, so don't despair if you don't have a daughter who isn't yet ready for this point. Your daughter will have to hold her wee long and not wake when her bladder shows that she needs to drain. It's best to wait until she's had dry nappies for many nights first.

Also, let her try to sleep without nappies. Shortly you will find out how ready it is. If it's evident after a few nights, she isn't prepared to stay dry, go back to her nappies at night, and don't make her feel like she has failed. Just tell her she's not ready yet, and she won't be long enough to try again. She's tall enough.

Don't be tempted to that the fluids of your baby. In the day, she will have six cups and eight cups. Do not offer her caffeine-containing drinks, including hot chocolate, shortly before bedtime. Caffeine will induce more weeks in the kidneys. If you ever wet your bed four or five years ago, see what you can do to make things easier for her. A night-light or potty can be any motivation to get up and down in her bed.

Try not to panic if your child takes a long time to stay dry at night. Bed weathering is considered natural for up to five years of age.

Your daughter, once days and nights, has achieved a lot, and let her know how well she has done. Give your friends and family leftover clothes or give them a nappy washing service with a friendly, happy wave of goodbye.

Many children are showing signs that they are ready to change from diapers to inside wear between 18 months and three years old, with girls usually start the transition a little earlier than boys.

HOW TO PREPARE YOUR GIRL AND MAKE TRAINING A LOT EASIER

One of the reasons girls should begin potty training earlier is that they reach an age at which they become more tolerant of soiling their pain fabric. When your daughter reaches this age, you may have already found that she was unhappy with her fall or that she needed to be adjusted in a particular way to you.

"Focus on the words you use." Here are 5 of our favorite tips for potty girls:

1. Teri Crane, the author of the famous toilet training book "Potty Train Your Child in Just One Day," says that adults should always interact in their language and schedules with their daughters about potty work. Crane told the Huggies diaper and pull-up business that many kids thought. In other words, you might think you're curious whether your daughter wants to go to the bathroom, whether she wants to step in, not whether she needs a toilet.

   Consider the vocabulary you use and understand that your daughter may take a while to understand what it means to "go to the bathroom."

2. According to Dr. Brown, parents need to be aware of when their daughter needs to go to the toilet because small girls tend to get a bladder infection if their daughter has a dirty pair of paint for a long time. The earlier you get your daughter into the bathroom, the better, so plan how much you and your child can go to the bathroom to see if she needs to go. Soon, your daughter will know that 20 minutes have passed since she went to the toilet, so it is time for us to go again.

3. Most little girls want their mom or caregiver to stay with them when they go to the bathroom, and you should never leave the child alone in the bathroom. FamilyDoctor.org, an American

Academy of Family Physicists website, recommended that adults read or talk to their daughters to make them relax and feel confident in the toilet. Many girls may end up feeling nervous or leaving the chair alone, and other small children may need help.

Consider the personality of your daughter before investing in toiletries.

4. Each child has its unique personality, and parents and guardians can first remember how their daughter learns before they go and buy various potty training devices. Each child has a unique personality. Many children feel awkward starting training in the adult toilet, so that families may choose to invest in a smaller, more child-friendly toilet than a removable seat. Tracy Marines, a Pennsylvania mom, told Parents.com that she often travels with Post-It notes when she has her daughter with her so that she can position the Post-It in public toilets with an auto sensor because auto-flush often scares your young daughter.

5. Nothing is higher than a positive attitude in the development of a child, and some potty training experts recommend that parents and guardians remain confident in the process of helping their children excel. According to the Mayo clinic, talking up-to-date and gently to your daughter on toilet training will help her realize that everybody is doing it and that she can master it. Reading potty training books and encouraging her–even when she does not go, though she felt she should be –are both ways to keep the experience positive. Take care to blame your daughter for an accident.

FamilyDoctor.org said parents should be patient and supportive when their child does not enter the bathroom in due course.

Recall that your daughter may take a few weeks or months to be fully educated. It is, therefore, crucial that your whole experience stays consistent and optimistic.

SECRETS TO POTTY GIRLS: HOW to POTTY TRAIN A GIRL FAST & EASY

Potty training girls Between 2 and 3 years of age, most of the girls show signs of potty training. They don't tuck a notebook underneath their arms, and after a substantial breakfast, they make a beeline to the toilet, but they are still ready. This does not mean smooth sailing from here–and clean undies. Potty girls is a challenge but learning certain tricks will help you to conquer the intestines!

The first phase of successful potty training is to ensure that the time is right– starting too early can only lead to failure; beginning late can make the process difficult. Search for signals that your daughter can't wet her pants anymore. Who are these? What are these? She can be involved in the shower, stay dry for long stretches, hang onto herself or pull up and down her pants.

You can continue once she shows these signs. Yet be assured you don't start with any other shift, not when a new babysitter comes in, not when a grandma is visiting, nor when you are on vacation.

Perhaps your daughter's battle with the potty isn't ready yet. Take the pail out and give it for a couple of weeks! Then try again for "hot."

REMEMBER, CHILDREN FROM OBSERVATION. You can do this in a few ways. To begin with, use the urge of your daughter to emulate you (as long as you are potty:-): she wants to be like mum and dad. Show her how you use the toilet to make her look around and promote copycat behavior. HAVING YOU HAVE THE PROPER EQUIPMENT. A child's potty is not just adorable; it's realistic. A small toilet helps to make kids feel much better than a large toilet. It's safer too–the rims of the full toilets encourage your child to go swimming unwittingly. You can also purchase an adjustable seat instead of purchasing a child-size potty. Just make sure it's tightly fastened and comfortable.

CULTIVATE COMFORT. Kids who feel confident in the toilet are much more likely to take potty training-make it clear from the beginning that a toilet is a special place for your baby. Enable it to be personalized with sticks or dry erase markers. And let her even practice where she sits on the toilet and pretends to go.

Most girls want to look beautiful–they dress up in flowy gowns and put on the shoes of their mother. This is another thing for potty-trained girls: take your daughter to the store and encourage her to select her most beautiful underwear. She would be much less likely than a bland pair last year to soil something she sees as exquisite or elegant.

KEEP CLEANLINESS IN MIND. Girls want to be clean in natural ways. They are much more aware that they sit in their filth than boys: they're questioning the doodie. So if you ask your daughter if she needs to go, she will probably be frank–she knows she makes her much happier by using the bathroom than peeing her pants in the middle of the reception room.

WIPE CORRECTLY. The act of wiping is a particular concern for girls-they must be advised to wipe from front to back to avoid the entry of germs in the bladder. Where boys are more vulnerable to "hot air," girls take special precautions. Probably, urinary tract infections in girls with toilet training are much more common than in other periods.

When your child finds it too difficult to understand the idea from front to back, encourage her to be dry. When she doesn't like cleaning–well, yeah, who's that? Consider purchasing toilet paper in different colors to encourage her to go. Journal of their favorite characters–T.P., too. Tweety Cat.

APPARATE TO Pee! Don't be shocked when your daughter takes her to the bathroom, but instead shakes outside the washing machine: she's at zoo number two, inside a canoe, or while shopping for shoes. She may be afraid to fall into the toilet and may not sit on it for long periods; she may also be constipated for several reasons.

Do not go back to slides while she demonstrates this behavior. Yeah, it's a lousy option (literally), but returning to slides could trigger potty regression. Instead, try to consider the viewpoint of your child and do what you can to help her resolve her worries (or her fiber intake).

And IT FUN Make fun with feces? It's a bit out, but making the cycle seem more like a journey and less like a mission will inspire your boy. You may use coloring for food to change the toilet watercolor or then reward it with something from a treasure box. You should read her favorite story when she's traveling or singing a song. Good it, and you're going to make it stick.

DON'T Forget Fantasy Children, who play doll-playing games and stuffed animals, are known to envision a household that has no pain bills. Play with her by showing her stuffed bear on the pot before going to winter. That reinforces the copycat behavior and solidifies the origin of the concept: it is nice to go to the bathroom in the morning.

Make a massive show of litter dances when your daughter pees into the potty, rejoice! When your daughter pees, rejoice! Recognize them if they piss in a bucket and not in their paints. Celebrate victories and good work. But don't get over the top – too many hoops will nervously deter your child from potty use.

PEE, PEE, AGAIN. Both children have injuries-it is not always something you first attempt to use the bath. However, the more your daughter uses the potty, the more she gets used to it. Be vigilant about clothes to support her along the way. Don't dress her in something that has too many buttons or too big an outfit.

TOILET TIPS AND TRICKS. It is good to get a pair of sleeves up in pursuit of the potty. Enable your child to accept naked (with no paintbrush, she will discover that she isn't faster attached to a toilet and a potty train).

Check for visual evidence (like jumping up and down or fidgeting) it needs to go.

Never blame or shame irrespective of your anger point. Retribution or embarrassment is the best way to avoid it.

Take a break if your daughter doesn't make progress. Then try again within a couple of weeks–you still have a chance before they're ready. When you don't go to the bathroom even after you have tried and tried again, ask for a doctor's aid.

It's entirely natural for a baby to become potty, yet to start soiling during the nap or sleeping hours.

LOOK AT NIGHTS DIFFERENTLY; Bedtime is bowel time to many children–about 15% of 5-years-olds and 10% of 6-year-olds already have bed accidents! The explanation is that sleeping takes a while to reinforce the connection between the brain and the bladder. You should still keep your child in a bedside diaper even after she is conditioned during the day, but you can drop the barrier once she wakes up in a row with a dry slide for several days.

The only thing to do by then is to put your kid in pain while she sleeps and makes her second wake up again. Too long a delay in growing can cause regression.

HOW TO POTTY TRAIN IN THREE DAYS ON YOUR SANITY

To potty train in three days in another world will be more straightforward: we will simply put our child's nose on their dirty windscreens and continuously say "no" before they have learned to use a toilet. We choose other paths in a civilized world. We beg. We do whatever we can to get our children to swap porcelain pampers. So we are still flooded with anger. Yet this is not the way it will be.

Potty training does not have to be a production process that lasts for as long as the mountain season (and feels wet): it can be carried out in three days.

You do need patience, perseverance, and potentially some carpet cleaner while taking the following measure.

But make sure your child is ready before you start. Only potty training lets you drain whether you are too young or too stubborn. When they display an interest in the bathroom, if they go on for long stretches without getting wet and can undress themselves, your child is probably ready.

THE Did Get!

Before you put this potty training approach into action step by step 3 days, you have to gather all your supplies. Other items you must have include a potty chair or a potty seat (to install one in both bathrooms), pants and socks, drinks (water or juice), and snacks for urination. You want a lot of cleaning supplies too–let's hear it for Lysol! –and towels to cover your car and furniture. Something that is consuming is going to do the trick.

DAY 1

If you want your child to train potty within three days, above all else, you will have to be consistent. Set aside a day when you're concentrating on flushing: a 3-day weekend or a week. Don't deviate entirely from the potty training plan and focus: just give pee and poop a piss.

To begin with, wear your child as soon as they wake up. You might think it's a big waste of money to put your child in underwear before they're potty trained; sure, you'd be right: pair after pair they'll ruin. Yet underwear becomes gross when it's damp and eventually dissuades your child from peeing. It'll be more productive if you put your kid in underwear with cartoon characters: Heaven forbids her to sponge Bob.

Next, tell them what you intend to do. Explain the potty point and why the diapers are safer. Place this thick on the first day, so that your child learns to equate a full bladder with loos.

Show them how the bathroom is used. Demonstrate what you need–clean, smooth, wash your face. First of all, children learn by observation.

Give them liquids, then. They have to use the bathroom to show your child how to use the bathroom. It is a safe way to make sure that they are packed with water and juice. When they have been prepared, put them on the pot at regular intervals–every 30-60 minutes–and keep them there even when they say they don't have to go. This means your child does not have to stay seated until Cosmo is read from front to back, but allows them to last for several minutes. Repeat this cycle all day long.

You may have to go more often, especially if you drink a lot. Look for signals that it is potty time and take them if they seem to be moving. They'll shower it with love every time they're right in the potty (and pee a lot from a drop to a bucket), hug them, cheer them on, give them five, tell them you're going to buy a BMW when they're sixteen (Don't worry, they'll forget). Don't threaten them or blame them if they're not doing it in time, just demonstrate that you're a little disappointed. Remind them carefully where the pee and the bag go (spoiler alert: the toilet!).

Tell your child that they need to go before you put your child down for a nap. (They'll say no if you ask.) You'll just want to put pressure on them as they sleep. Most children stay wet even though they are dry during waking hours.

DAY 2

On the second day, a lot of the first is replicated. It also has its problem, however, because not all children acclimatize as fast as you hoped. If that is the case, remember that things happen: even though your child takes fish to the toilet, they fall sometimes. Many children get distracted and forget about it. Others prefer to pee in the cupboard. Yet if your kid uses the bathroom even more often than the living room robbery, you know that they are improving.

Reward them too because they remain dry. Children respond to rewards (after all, they are human only). But, every time you go to the bathroom, you reward them: unexpectedly, at every meal, your child demands plums.

Instead, reward them for staying dry, meaning that they get a bonus if they deserve it and not because they claim to be.

Spend the second day reinforcing the lessons learned from the first day and searching for exploitation. Many kids keep soiling in the hope of putting them in a paintbrush (which is, actually, more convenient for them). But don't give up anything. You will outsmart the wee in this war of wits.

DAY 3

Follow the trends on the last day and take your child out of the house. You don't have to go far— the nearest park or café. The goal here is to encourage you to use the bathroom before you go home. You also know that toilets are not always close by – you have to control your bladder for a little longer before you hit it.

Day 3 means further conversations with your child about the importance of toilet training, but it is also essential to show how far they have come.

Celebrate their accomplishments, however insignificant. Kids love and respond like ego-maniacs to affection.

Not each kid trains potty on the first attempt (or the first twenty). When you lose the fight, admit defiance. Then try again in a few weeks–you still have a chance before they're ready. But to try again doesn't mean that you never try. You will finally teach your child potty. When you don't, in the mid-50s, they can live in your cellar.

If they're still not talking to the toilet after you've tried and tried again, seek the help of a pediatrician.

A NOTE ABOUT NIGHTS. As described above, children can not always regulate their bladders while they sleep: when it comes to training potty, sleep is a bummer. You will know that it is time for your child to wear napkins and night slides when their sleep slides stay dry a few days in a row. It can happen a few days or weeks after a good day. Perhaps it could take a few months. Kids wet the bed until they are six years old–about 15% of five-year-olds and 10% of those six-year-olds will still be affected by bed incidents. It's not that they're naughty–it's natural! The relation between the brain and the bladder is not good enough to alert them when they have to go. It is necessary to remove the diaper of your child as soon as they wake up (both morning and nap). When you leave it too long, there is a chance that they will regress. You'll go back to the fact that you're in a portable toilet and you'll quickly use it.

Finally, potty training is a pain in the ass. And after that, risks remain: the times they have to go would be painful. In the middle of the night: perhaps. In a packed restaurant: definitely. Ten minutes after you've left your house for a two-hour road trip: yeah, that's a sure thing. Yet it gets simpler the older a child is. Going to the toilet is normal, and your kid won't even worry about it twice one day long.

Do you want your girl to be educated in 1 or 3 days?

It is another joy to have a baby girl. Five Examples of Potty Training. For Girls, She could have inherited your hair, or she might have had the dimples of your husband. This way, she'll be the family queen. Yet, learning potty is one thing that can not be inherited. So what are the five ways girls should train potty?

Above all, a little girl is easier to train because she can do what is needed by looking at her mother as an example. Your baby girl must be taught potty, not only by setting an example but also by daily training. Girls generally sit in the toilet bowl to piss and shit. First of all, tell her how to sit on the potty. You should take her to the potty after that and ask her to do what you just have done. Do not press her and ensure that she is sitting safely to prevent accidents.

Second, use an alternative if your explanation has failed. Use a potty doll to reassure her that she will go to the bathroom anytime she wants to. Switch the doll to the doll and make it look like it is being used by the doll. This is going to attract your daughter's attention as toys and dolls are her playtime companion. She treats her toys as her children, and she will please her children, and she will do what she will to do and use the potty.

Third, your daughter's clothes will be beautiful and comfortable. This would make it easier for her to go to the toilet and take care of her bathroom needs. Nothing should work for the same purpose as wearing a shirt. Ask her to clean from front to back to prevent spreading bacteria.

Fourth, consider the readiness or willingness of your daughter. Often she displays the expression of her face and her excitement and says that she needs to use the potty. In doing so, it is easier for her to use the pot daily without too much effort, time, and money. We will then have daily urination and balanced bowel movements.

Fifth, motivation in potty training is often present. Your daughter won't take action or help in potty training without that. Recall that your persuasive words are also beneficial. A mildly compelling cheer or expression can make a significant difference from doing nothing. Convince her to use the potty from time to time, and perhaps she will. Keep in mind that it will never push you for that is something other than convincing.

Now that you know the five ways girls can train potty, start with your daughter. Don't waste any minute because it's fantastic to see that your little princess has already learned to use the bowl.

POTTY GIRLS TRAINING — USING INSIDER KNOWLEDGE

Potty girls are the same as a boy's training. Still, you, mom or dad, can motivate your girl to work more thoroughly with the girl's potty exercise by using small information.

For example, in general, women are often social creatures (yes, there are exemptions), and you would like to take notice and use this to your advantage if your little potty trainee falls into this class.

For starters, if you remain alongside her during the toilet training phase, she will probably cooperate with you more fully. It's quick to do. Keep her potty chair in your house, even in the kitchen, in the mainstream of activities.

Many families have several potty chairs to make it easier for a child to find one, especially at the start of the toilet training.

If your kid sits on her potty, don't leave her alone to work on it. Take a stack of books and have a good time reading together. Use a small tray together with color. Singing songs and playing finger together.

The keyword here is "together." Potty-separated girls often make things harder than they have to be.

Here is another way to use the instincts of your daughter to support her with potty training. Enhance the therapeutic skill of your daughter with her favorite doll or invest in a unique potty training doll that she may "train" to use a potty chair.

She will enjoy helping her doll in this way, and you will have the added advantage of knowing how much she knows the toilet exercise by listening to the updates that she sends her doll.

Besides, make it easy for your child to move to clothe. Dresses are fabulous and tend to be a good potty option because they don't have to be separated from the potty chair, but the thickness of the fabric will make it hard for a kid to take his dress off the road–and in a rush.

If your daughter selects a handful of appropriate clothes, she will feel much more comfortable and interested in keeping her garments dry and clean.

If your home is noisy or disturbing, it may not be a good time for potty training now, whether you have a girl or a boy. Children must concentrate on what they are expected to know, and as a parent, it is wise to relax their households during their preparation.

Use a potty training chart to keep your kid informed and encouraged. Enable her to choose stickers on the map. Holding a second chart for her potty doll will also help keep her interested.

Here the bottom line? When you spend some time thinking about things in your little girl's interest and consider her unique personality, you will build potty ideas customized to her needs.

Remember that she loves validation will allow you to stay calm and patient and listen to your suggestions.

Thinking outside the box will help you enjoy the benefits beyond the usual stickers and sweets (for example, when our fresh undies stay dry all week). Potty training for girls is about thinking about what is best for your daughter and about working on the practical aspects of toiletries for her benefit.

All you need to learn about Girls ' Small Education- is it easier?

Potty girls ' training can be a tough time if she refuses or does not obey the directions. The girl will be hesitant to use the potty, has accidents, or do not want to use the potty. Although that sounds natural, issues will occur in the future if the problem is not correctly resolved. During potty training for children, the following are essential tips.

1. You must use a method that works for many other parents. Because it is easier to teach potty girls than boys, your time could be wasted and your girl worse. Unless the approach you use is unsuccessful, it will be much harder.

2. When your girl refuses your orders, you need to know how to respond. Therefore, it is so crucial at the right moment to know what to say. As long as you fail, your suggestions will have less effect in the future. It is because your girl should feel more energetic and responsive to your orders.

3. Constipation can be a concern, and you have to respond accordingly. This may be the most challenging part of girls ' potty training, as they feel they can not release.

4. Knowing what to say in a tough situation for your child. Some girls can scream, yell, run, or even hit when they try not to use the potty. It is genuine, and you must use the correct words to calm them down. It's exceptional to be 18 months old and three years old.

When you are like some parents and believe your girl can use the potty, the following adverse effects must be considered.

1. Health problems can occur if girls ' potty training is completed too late. Do you know the disorder known as retentive encopresis? This happens because of untreated constipation issues and starts between the ages of 3 and 4. The disease causes the lower intestines to stretch or even tear. The effect is swollen, hard stools and bowel movements are not possible.

This can lead to other disorders, such as mega-colon and bladder infections.

2. If girls don't do potty training early enough, psychological issues may occur. Children may be mocked or humiliated at daycare or pre-school in their friends' group. That is because many other kids can no longer use disposable slides.

3. Girls ' potty training gets more robust as they get older. This is because they rely more on disposable slides and find it hard to adjust. Potty girls ' training will take place as early as 18 months.

4. For each year they decide to use disposable diapers, you can spend an additional 2000 dollars on paint supplies. You must also feed neglectful global slide corporations that plan to use slides for as long as possible.

5. Disposable slides contribute significantly to the waste landfill that society today faces and harms the environment.

6. Girls ' potty training takes a small fraction of the time per month compared to changing slides. This takes a tremendous amount of time and can be avoided.

Girls ' Potty Training-5 Great tips for helping your little one use the Potty!

Potty girls ' training can be a bit overwhelming work for many parents who want to make the job so easy as they can but do not know how to get started. Thankfully, statistics show that it is generally easier for girls to train than small boys, but it can still be challenging to learn when to start and exactly what to do.

Overall, correctly done, potty training can be fun and rewarding and can not be frustrating at all.

Below are five tips to continue the cycle well:

1. Make sure your girl is ready to learn the potty. Some children continue to use the potty as early as 18 months, while others maybe three years old. The cycle must not be speeded up too soon as studies indicate that children must be ready before training starts.

2. Put your child in the pot and make her feel confident with it. Spend some time before the training begins to let your kid know that there is nothing to fear, which encourages her to become a good girl with the potty.

3. Teach your little one when she has finished the right way to clean. Wiping from front to back is necessary to prevent infection of the urinary tract.

4. Reward your little girl for her excellent performance and celebrate her achievement. A perfect way to do so is to show other family members how well they do with stickers on a map. Reinforcement and affirmation are essential when your small toilet is being educated.

5. Treat them gently and lovingly without raising the voices when injuries occur. Understand from the outset that this is a wonderful opportunity for you both, and those good days and bad days will be there. Only go back to the usual routine without responding when an incident happens, and she is comfortable.

Mass training for girls can be a way to get both parent and child together and can be a way that gives your little girl a great sense of accomplishment as she learns to regulate the bowel and bladder. There is so more you can do to make your little girl's transition from nappies to underpants a positive experience.

POTTY TRAINING: GIRLS CAN BE DIFFERENT FROM BOYS

One of the key reasons why girls are taught potty by their mothers can be in almost any situation. And because girls and moms use the toilet the same way, it is fair for the girls to learn the art of the potty much faster.

During potty training for children, there can be many tricks and methods, and mothers should learn as many things as possible as the time for the practice will be very limited if the methods are correctly administered. Several things to remember: when a mother uses the bathroom, invite the daughter to get to know the procedure.

Dress your daughter in loose clothes when practicing potty so that you get to it quickly and easily.

When possible, send the girl with her father and brother to the toilet when she starts to wonder and then attempts to go the same direction as the males in the room. Confusion is not an excellent training feature.

Sitting the dolls on the potty and hearing stories about how the dolls go to the toilet can also be a learning experience because girls will take the same places as their dolls.

Rewards will also support her when she was.

In addition to strategies and tricks at starting the process of children, parents should be told to teach hygiene and the correct way to clean their daughter. Wiping from front to back is suggested as the medically correct procedure because it minimizes the exposure to bacteria that helps to prevent infection. Potty-training illnesses and diseases are the last things you want to encounter as a parent.

Knowledge is beneficial for parents, not only through tips for potty training for children, but also health and hygiene.

When to Train Your Girl is the same method of potty training for both boys and girls? So what're the gaps if not? When do you teach the girls potty? The main difference is that while urinating boys are a little messy than girls and the main concern for girls is hygiene so that the earlier you start girls with proper toilet hygiene habits, the better.

Before beginning your girl with potty training, make sure she is trained physically and mentally, so the girl does not feel as if she is being forced to use the potty. The signs that your girl is eager to begin potty training are a facial expression or signs of distress when she needs to go potty, stay dry for about two hours, and to go to the toilet. Also, make sure there are no other stress factors in the family, such as traveling, waiting, or getting a baby and major illness or death in the family.

Whenever you see that your girl is ready to begin potty training, you have to determine what terms you should use in public, and then you will buy your girl a potty chair. Get your girl used to the potty chair and sit on it for around five minutes at regular intervals, when she gets used to it, recommend that you take it with you to the bathroom when she says she wants to go. Try to compliment your girl and be positive when it is good.

Girls are typically not hard to train as the boys are generally messy while they are urinating. The biggest issue with girls is hygiene, so it is essential to begin teaching girls hygiene early, first of all, to let them know that the toilet seat is dry does not mean that any germs make first to wipe off the place before they sit. Once the potty has been applied, instruct them to wash from front to back to prevent contamination and advise them to paddle rather than to wash hard. Try to use the softest tissue you can afford as much as possible, which is gentle on the skin.

Tips for Potty Training-Children!

Here are some precious tips for potty training, boys! Number one-if you're working on potty training for your child-leave, the dad out without you. I know most modern women believe their husbands are like hairy women but don't fool themselves. If your husband's answer is entirely truthful, I will guarantee that most men claim they have a feeling of awkward toilet training for their daughter.

In the practical sense, it can be tough to ask men to teach a girl to clean, for example. They may be confused about the way to clean or where to start- from front to back or from front to front. Because of the essence of a guy, he's probably not going to ponder about too much and let your daughter find it out. For hygienic purposes, however, wiping from back to front may lead to infection, so your child must be taught right from the beginning. Your husband would probably not know this unless he is qualified as a pediatrician or pediatric nurse.

Certain people can't cope with child-raising activities, including clothing change and potty training. To order to prevent needless friction between you and your boyfriend, girls should not pressure the situation with the most realistic potty training tips. On the other hand, today, many people are very relaxed, changing the diapers of their infant. When your husband doesn't, he doesn't suggest something is wrong with him. I'm just trying to make you conscious for all who are, that maybe he can't handle this situation very well. Many people are uncomfortable in coping with these jobs. While it does not want to discuss this with you, it may still cause needless anxiety. When he finds himself holding those images outside his potty training course, he may begin to doubt his own mental and sexual health. Again, this doesn't mean your friend has psychological issues, but people don't want to be pushed into awkward circumstances.

On the other hand, most men have no issue when asked to help potty boys train because they can quickly identify with their friend; that is, they know how all parts work, and there is little risk that a girl will become contaminated after inadequate cleaning. Now, let's take it from the little girl. Little girls assume that their fathers and their mother are different, but they clearly don't understand or know how they are. Obviously, with their daughters, fathers can not illustrate how they use the toilet as mothers can, but their sons definitely can.

The best potty training tips, ladies, honestly are not to push your husband or daughter into a circumstance that he or she is unhappy with or that may lead to potential stress. If you find him trying to help his daughter with his toilet training, then leave him alone. He decides for himself if the situation is secure. If he doesn't, he will probably call you for help, and you will go to his rescue with compassion. When your husband is happy with the situation, your daughter would certainly.

How should not your girl have to be so painful?

For most parents, Potty girls or boys-babies-don't expect something. After all, who wants to deal with filthy clothing-and even rugs, bikes, tables, etc.-?

Although the problem may have additional problems of fear and uncertainty for new parents, even experienced parents fear the idea.

Luckily, teaching kids how to use a child's potty seat or kid's toiled seat doesn't have to be as complicated and painful as other parents assume. In general, potty training for girls appears to take place earlier than for boys. I don't know what to say to all of you chauvinists, except that it's well known. Girls seem to be able to grow this ability much faster than boys for some reason.

Part of the explanation may be that boys will learn two "modes." Urinating for boys is not the same as knowing the Number 2 Protocol. As many parents know, few boys can tell the difference between them when they need to relieve themselves. They only need to be moving. Therefore, boys must not   only learn two different skills but also learn the difference of what they experience–even though what feels like an' natural' urine needs could be urinating

POTTY TRAINING FOR GIRLS-THE THREE MOST COMMON APPROACHES

Potty training is an enjoyable activity and a milestone in a child's life. The reason many parents experience the opposite is that they don't plan properly and work with a validated process. In this post, I'll help you approach potty training in the right way and prevent all dissatisfaction from the beginning. Once it's time to train your little girl, it's essential that you first pick the method before you do anything else. Once you have selected a process, planning for the big day is much more comfortable. The three most common methods of potty training for girls are discussed in this report.

1. **The "nudist" method:** This method is cheap and straightforward but very uncomfortable. Any or two pots are added, and the child is allowed to walk naked for 3-7 days after describing the pots. There will be many incidents, and the goal is to raise awareness about kindergarten functions. The kid will soon discover all by himself that using the potty is much more convenient than getting stuff down the leg. I can only support this approach if one of the two methods below could not be obtained.

2. **The "potty routine" method:** This approach deals with repetition and repetitive learning. The timer is used, and the child has been taken to the potty for around three days at set times (e.g., once an hour and after meals). The child will quickly learn what's expected of the parent during the potty time with instruction from the adult, and within one or two days, she will know what to do when she wants help without a timeout. It is a very successful tool, but it takes time.

3. This method is a little more expensive but by far the most popular for girls (because it uses a special weeding doll). **Dr. Phil's One Day method.** The underlying principle behind this approach is that teaching is the best way to know something. Through training the doll to use the potty, the kid easily teaches himself. After this technique was seen on Dr. Phil several years ago, it has been both boy's and girls ' best-known tool for potty training.

Though the approach of the first is the preferred method for potty training for girls, choosing the way you think best matches your child's circumstances is essential.

What's the fastest way to get a girl to Potty Train?

As a baby, I always told parents that the effectiveness of potty training depends heavily on the readiness and encouragement of their daughter to go or not to the pot. Most children age and mature differently, but as soon as they are able, you should not teach them the etiquette of the bathroom.

Research has also shown that some girls start as early as 17-18 months, while others might not be ready until four years old. If you want to know when to start potty training, you should note that most parents tend to start with girls between the ages of two and three, which is the age at which you start.

Furthermore, experience has shown that girls typically can be trained more quickly than boys, and many of them are ready about three months earlier in comparison with boys.

To get things going, I managed to train most kids through the purchase of potty training equipment and concentrate at most 1-2 strategies. Keeping this in mind, you should first buy your girl a pot and tell her it's her own. I always stress the purchasing of a real pot, not a toiler adaptor, as both girls and boys at that age may look frightening. Make sure it's stylish, so it doesn't look like a boys ' potty.

Once it comes to how to potty a child, you will find a way to inspire her to use the equipment that is freshly purchased.

There are many ways to do this now, so we should focus on watching and learning. When you see that your daughter uses the toilet every day, she soon discovers that this is a natural part of life, because children always want to do whatever adults do. This will serve as a motivating factor, given that with age, your daughter will begin to dislike the feeling of dirty.

Motivation is also one of the best potty girls ' training tips. Just speak to her and let her know how important it is and how fun it is to go to the potty, too (hint: give her something to do, read, paint or watch television). Many girls will take a long time to complete so they can get bored and therefore have something fun to do.

Based on all outlined so far, I would tell from my observations that inspiration would help young girls go very far so that they can also realize how necessary the potty is and motivate them to use it.

Until you begin, however, make sure your child is ready for potty training and is of the right age (18 months to 3/4 years).

Was Potty Patty a girl's favorite way to train potty?

What exactly is your child's best way to train potty? Should you cultivate and allow you to use your toilet instead of your diapers? And maybe it's the song that made Look Who's Talking Too famous when the parents sang, "You have to fight for a potty right!" Probably not. No, the perfect way to teach your daughter is in today's hectic world in the form of an adorable, anatomically correct doll called Potty Patty.

The one-day Potty Patty Doll and Potty Training system were celebrated as a cure for parental potty training. The popular method will teach your child to use the potty for a maximum of 2 weeks in one day!

The Potty Training In One Day (PTIOD) system underlines the approach of "learning to teach" is a way to give the child the trust not to use paint strips anymore. Your child is the one who tells Potty Patty to use the toilet, and your child is the one who benefits from knowing. Your kid plays with the doll with such optimistic reinforcement, when both girls say farewell to their "big day" slides. Potty patty packages The software provides all the necessities to train your child in the potty. Potty shoes, a comfortable training pad, the Potty Patty doll, and a very informative book and DVD are also available.

This curriculum builds on the progress and trust of your child. The method is easy, productive, and straightforward. PERIOD is intended for parents who are unsure about the potty training process, scared, and reluctant. You and your child will realize with the system and the Potty Patty doll that you are not alone.

The 3 Step Method

The 3 Step Method is a quick, stress-free method that brings your child in only one day from diaper to the pot. The first stage is the evaluation and planning process. Parents are encouraged to know if their child is ready for their "Big Day" by reading an awareness guide. The guide stresses that your child will never get educated if he or she is not ready.

The second stage is very much the case. It is about the "Big Day," when your kid says good-bye to clothes and introduces itself socially to the potty. This is where the one-day Potty Training Program makes all the difference. Your kid isn't pressured only to use the potty here; instead, she teaches her potty doll and learns to use the potty herself in that way. This is an excellent loop of motivation, constructive bonding and teamwork.

The third and last step is the follow-up stage, in which unavoidable incidents are dealt with. Instead, mistakes never undo the "Big Day" of your kid; they are opportunities to improve the potty Patty training lessons. Here, repetition is a primary priority.

10 TIPS TO POTTY TRAIN A GIRL

Small training will begin when your child is ready for physical, mental, and social work in all three areas. Your child must be able to take the appropriate measures. You should understand how the body works and know the clues.

They will always want to know.

If your child has a potty chair and knows how to switch from slides to pants, remind them to bring their favorite "pet" or stuffed animal for you. Let them first teach their "kid." This means they understand the process and can continue. If you find it complicated, you may want to put it off, but if they are willing to try, go ahead and think about implementing it.

This is an exciting yet also stressful time for both you and your girl, I can tell you from experience. It's a step away from childhood, and for both of you, that will be a relief. Changing diapers isn't something that most of us want to do. I will send you a few tips because I have already been through this phase twice.

1) **Watching Mom:** It is a practice that they will have to try to grasp, however humiliating it may be. If you see them, they get their idea much quicker than if you tried to get them to sit on the potty chair.

2) **Show the Chair of Potty**: You'll want to do a lot of things on this page. Show the infant the chair, and instruct the "poor girls" to use it instead of slides. Because she has already seen you if she feels the need to go, she will have an idea of what to do.

3) **Undies "poor girl":** Make this case a landmark. Take her to the section of children and let her choose what she wants. It could be a Disney character or a Film, but she can choose it. I recall how happy our girls were when they revealed their choices.

4) **Injuries Happen:** Injuries not only occur but also occur at the most inconvenient time possible. Be prepared with both a device for cleaning (fresh socks, etc.) and the courage to handle it with grace.

5) **Correct Development Stage:** No matter what your baby books tell you, a child will be ready if she's ready for potty training. This is on its schedule, not yours or others. To move it too early can be detrimental.

6) **Bathroom Fears:** while not familiar, some kids are terrified of public bathrooms. Many children have vast spaces, and sounds echo. Don't just write it off if your child shows proof of this fear. Find out what's troubling them, then work at a time. Maybe you want to find public toilets that are at first a little more child-friendly.

7) **Talk to the pediatrician:** The doctor of your child can be beneficial to this. The doctor will inform you that the child is ready to look for it. The doctor will also help you deal with the bathroom's anxiety.

8) **Celebrate success but don't punish failure:** It may take some time for full control to remove both urine and feces. Each time the child makes it to the chair, cheer. Nevertheless, don't want to blame them because he or she slept profoundly and waters the room. It can also build a fear of doing so, and this is not good for the health of the infant.

9) **Books:** A variety of children's potty training books are now available. Read them with your child so that you can reinforce what you have discussed.

10)   **Breaking the habit of the potty chair:** Teach them to use the "tall" potty until your child has control. You will need a paddle at first, as most toilets are too large to get on with a small child comfortably. Perhaps you want to take some of the same steps to make this transition.

Although it's not always easy, it is undoubtedly a good milestone when your daughter can "go" alone at last. This will be a relatively quick move with your diligence.

The principle of one day's training

It is to spend an entire day teaching your child without interruption. I clarified that they showed signs that they were happy and old enough to step into standard underwear. I gave my daughter some lightly salted popcorn and her first coke, which would support us one day with our potty training! Some smart children can want to extend it for many more days just to obtain these treatments! I made her sit 10 minutes on a pot and kept her occupied with books, toys, etc. She was able to eat some popcorn after ten minutes, drink her soda, and play for another 10. At this time, we held her out of slippers, pull-ups, or socks, yes, that means that the ground half is open. Then we started again, sat on a pot for 10 minutes, and then increased our time off the potty every time for around five to ten minutes. So you will start with 10 minutes, 10 minutes off, 15 minutes off, 10 minutes off, 20 minutes off, etc. Continuing to load them with her snack to get them hungry, the more chances they drank to play. You can drink or snack, but this was my favorite day for this particular day!

Once you've started potty training, buy multiple pairs of underwear with the favorite character of your kid. Wrap them in beautiful paper or give them a special presentation. Know that your child has had some excellent potty training and is ready for underwear with his favorite character. Then after they model them and put them on, clap and do a lot, remind them that Cinderella does not like to get wet or dirty (replace her favorite name with the person). Don't forget, run fast to keep them dry and clean as soon as you have to go to the toilet. Some of my friends attempted this when they realized that their children were ready for company, understood, and were still too busy to play. When they have an incident, this message (or e-mail) may be attempted.

Dear one (the name of the child), I am so proud of you that I know how to use the potty! I'm also glad that you've had some underwear in my photo. Seek to keep your parents in mind as soon as you feel the urge to go to the bathroom. Please remember I don't want to get dirty or wet, and when I'm dry, I love it!

Sometimes we all have incidents, and if you do, please tell your parents immediately! They're not going to be mad, and then they can easily wash them, clean them up, and wear them.

I'm proud of you!

Note that every child grows differently. The age range can be between 18 months and three years. At 4, the majority of children are entirely autonomous.

If you begin to understand that your child is not ready, try again in a couple of months.

You can not complete potty training for your child until they are ready. You can start the preparation, but when it finishes, they decide. It isn't a war, and if it starts to go that way, put it off. Usually, toilet training can not be carried out in one day. You can do a lot to get the basics down, but plan and be prepared for injuries, should they happen.

Include an additional pair of clothing, a plastic bag to store wet wipes and wet wipes in the vicinity. Do not yell, threaten, or condemn if an incident happens.

Bad weather is natural. The nighttime took a lot longer for both guys. We used night pulls at bedtime and would try every couple of months a few nights in a row.

Dryness at night is only accomplished when the body of a child is created. This can't be "taught," because it's not a talent. I know many boys who kept wearing pulls until the age of seven and eight. I asked our pediatrician, and they recommended that the doctor have it up to remove issues, but that individual child might not develop this capacity until later.

POTTY GIRLS TRAINING TIPS HOW DO YOU HANDLE YOUR DAUGHTER TO GO POTTY?

Below are some ideas you should take into account.

You never want to frighten your daughter or to give her a toilet training rejection. For this, it is essential to plan for her great day.

Buy the necessary materials two weeks before the class. Essential supplies for preparation include potty, pants and wipes. You may want to take your daughter with you and let her pick the things she wants. She might choose to use a pink potty, for example. She can also wear pink flower-designed training pants. Bring her with you to make the use of these products easy.

Equip your mind with essential toilet training knowledge. You can ask experienced parents for any tips, or you can choose to read self-help posts.

Show the potty and let your daughter play with it. It will encourage her to become acquainted with the potty. You should even pretend to play with her. For example, imagine you're going to teach her doll potty. Let the doll sit on the pot and tell your child that she'll do the same early.

Always remind your daughter of the big day ahead. On the night before the potty training, tell her it's a beautiful day tomorrow because she will be a fantastic girl. Feel excited about her. On the training itself, you should always be concentrated and relaxed.

On the first day of training, remember that today's big day is your baby. A lack of attention can result in your daughter's adverse reactions.

Make sure all the correct materials are ready. Place them in an available area.

Put on training pants for your daughter and encourage her to drink a big glass of milk or tea.

Use a quick timer. Ensure sure your daughter goes every 15 minutes to the potty.

Prepare yourself for injuries. Don't blame your daughter if a mishap happens. Remind her gently that in the potty, she will pee or shower and not in her underwear.

Thank your daughter for every achievement. Let her believe she's doing a good job. You will relax her further by offering her favorite candy or some fun stickers.

Don't make trouble. Continue your good beginning until your daughter is sufficiently educated. Make the appropriate modifications depending on how easily your daughter understands.

You have it; the efficient ways to train your toilets. Potty workouts shouldn't be bad for you and your kids. You will excel by being patient and concentrated, and by using fun strategies to get your child's attention. Who knows, in 1-3 days you will produce good results!

Patience and compassion are essential for the business of potty training. When your child is curious and willing to learn the procedure, the next thing to do is give your girl full attention and your particular time. To teach your daughter effectively and to see fast results, here are a few helpful tips.

• Allow her the ability to observe and learn. Children know what they see in their world as they mimic it. In this respect, the first thing you need to do is to prove that you use the toilet. Even your daughter is more likely to use your toilet when she sees that her parents, father, and some friends use the toilet at school. This is where you need to be to help. This may be a mess, but teach her how to clean up.

- Provide the correct equipment and resources available for training. There are smaller pots you can purchase that will give you complete safety than using a full-size toilet. Check to ensure that the devices are strong and stable before purchasing the equipment.

- The right dress to wear is part of proper toilet training for children. Your option would either achieve or break your objective to teach her how to use the toilet as quickly as possible. When you have agreed to get rid of the painting, you don't want to go back with it because things have happened to try and turn it into a potty. Any effort you have made otherwise will all be thrown away.

Useful toilet training tips are available to girls that are very helpful in teaching your child how to use the toilet. Keep investigating and selecting the right methods for you and your kids.

Most kids are willing to please parents and caregivers, so they are usually cooperative in potty education. They are going to do their premature dance, you're going to say they're going to the bathroom, and they're golly going to do it! However, not all children are versatile or compliant. Some are utterly angry and defiant. A parent who answers with his / her anger and resentment can derail potty training.

The first thing that a child should avoid toilet training is to reassess the developmental maturity of the infant Remember even a child's age. By the age of 3, except for disability, most children are old enough to start toilet training.

Test your actions next. Are you flawlessly consistent? If you quit the working dog, you may be tempted to abandon that night's training. When you do, the growth of your child will be delayed or completely sidetracked. Are you obvious or confusing? If you save time in a rush by putting your baby in hurts, not shoes, then you send out mixed signals. This undermines your success, which unnecessarily makes your child feel like a failure.

But let's say that your child is ready physically. So we can presume you have consistent and clear expectations. Also, children should avoid using the toilet rather than their pants. Some children are like that. Others are simpler to use, versatile, and adaptable, and some are more adaptable. Not so. More so.

Then there are a handful of entirely stubborn children. Many children are battling for everything and everything–the potty time is no exception. I saw children staring at the eye of their parents, confidently saying, "No, I don't have to pee," while urine is flowing down their hands, socks and shoes! (Not a pretty picture, but a practical part of kindergarten) As it is tenting to retaliate in nature, the power fight will escalate with a loud, angry parent response. The entire toilet learning cycle is complex, unpredictable, and attractive. Let me be explicit here unmistakably. I never met a kid co-operating in potty training unless he was scoffing, teasing, calling a "baby," or crying endlessly. Uncontrolled rage does not inspire children; it morter their walls of frustration and mistrust. Physical and verbal violence alienates children and scares them. Abuse, particularly from loved ones, steals children's confidence and self-esteem. The uncontrolled rage of a parent teaches a lot, but nothing constructive or fruitful.

And how do I advise parents to react to resistance? First, relax as a child slowly warms up to the toilet idea. Live as calm and relaxed as you can. Resist heavy-handedness and force a showdown. A highly charged loop of power struggles can be lit when parents pressure a child over interest or speed too hard, or too quickly. Be mindful of your desires and aspirations, but always listen politely to the concerns of your kids. Don't encourage your child to yell or hit you, but support him as much as you can with a good spirit and a positive attitude.

So here's a tip from a colleague who has recently been in power struggles for months. Out of sheer desperation, she just sat down and felt sorry for some children battling control overall — it's not an exception.

She told her she knew how hard it was to learn how to use the potty, but she was sure she could. The three-year-old girl was pleased to learn that her mom knew that it was difficult for her to master the bathroom. Something shifted until she believed her mother recognized her disappointment. Once her anxiety and concerns were talked about freely, she was much more positive and comfortable with the potty.

But not all power struggles just stop. If a child is temperamentally unstable, or upset at actual or imaginary accidents (like sibling rivalry), children may be stubborn and refuse to use potty — even if they're about to burst! If you say, "Do you have to sweetheart, sweetie?" They're going to yell, "NOOOOO!" These people even kick and launch themselves into a blossoming tantrum!

There is too much room for defiance for questions that require "yes" or "no." So when it comes to battling a potty problem, children still win. We can't make children keep their urine or bowels, after all. We will also inspire them to do so with motivation and consequences.

For demanding or reluctant children, consistently and honestly say, "It is time to try to get potted right now." Let go of your voice at the end of the sentence instead of going up. It's straightforward; it gives more trust and shows you mean business. Tell your child he doesn't have to potty, just sit down and stand on the toilet. (Say this ONCE; otherwise, you end up with a two-year-old harangue!) When you talk, extend your hand gently to enable your child to make its way into the potty. Show appreciation by providing the right option for developments: "When you try, do you want privacy or want me nearby?" If a child doesn't go after five to ten minutes, let her pull her pants, thank her for the effort, and allow her to try again later.

When your child still fights with you, use the quiet moments to remind her that it's your responsibility to encourage her to use the pot. Listen and accept her questions and suggestions, no matter how dumb they sound. Let your child know that you need his assistance and support to be a good mother or dad. So note he should be proud to be a good assistant, so learn to use the bathroom.

When your child is four or older and still not qualified in the bathroom, practical assistance from outside the family is needed. When power struggles are persistent or if they are abusive, it may be a call for help from the child or a symptom of some underlying issue. If so, turn to a competent child psychologist for assistance. (Many local agencies charge an income-based sliding fee.) Monitor your extreme reactions as well. Turn to a family therapist or psychologist for support when you hit the end of the rope.

Solutions can be shed light only on a few sessions.

You may also turn to seasoned individuals, such as grandparents, childcare providers and friends who have children educated in the toilet, who know your child well. Your fresh ideas can be especially helpful if you are in the midst of power struggles. The following toilet training books can also be helpful.

ERRORS IN POTTY TRAINING

Beyond the usual fear of pooping on the toilet, children just don't get used to sitting on a stool, so it may be hard for them to get hanging from it. Help keep your child's body going by giving him plenty of fluids and fruits and vegetables loaded with nutrients. This would make it easier to go to the toilet. When you note any significant changes in the daily behavior of your child (say he used to poop once a day, and now he isn't pooping), discuss the constipation remedies with your child's doctor. Your doctor may also want to see your child so that there is no other underlying issue. "Often, it just takes a few days to back the training and get your child on track," says Dr. Klemsz.

After all, a child can be upset by potty training, which can cause constipation and eventually discomfort as it poops.

Take the time, "The framework, potty or toilet, and help must be given, but your child must want to do it," says Dr. Klemsz. So note, if your child has a lot of stress (such as a recent transfer or a new brother), it will speed up potty training. However, as long as you offer potty training, "for most babies, they'll have a fair shot," says Dr. Klemsz. In the meantime, she gives this sound advice: "Instead of looking at potty training as a challenge, see it as an opportunity for your child to get to know him better— how he learns and how he adapts to stress. You will learn a great deal about the temperament of your child, and the lessons you will learn about your child through potty training will educate her about other challenges.

The risks of early potty training.

There are many reasons why your child should be trained as early as possible. You want to avoid purchasing slides; they're environmentally harmful, costly, and disgusting. You want your child to be in front of the game. There are no-brainer explanations for early potty training. However, in contrast to the size of the reasons you should not, the reasons why you want to train your child early on sound dumb.

According to Dr. Steve Hodges, MD. from the BedwettingAndAccidents.com website, the willingness of children under the age of three to take full responsibility for their toilet activities is irrational.

How can early potty training possibly go wrong?

Of course, children will undergo potty training well in advance of their age of three, but will they do it properly? (Yes, the right way.) When it comes to using the potty, a mistake can lead to some health issues.

Dr. Hodges states that from the approximately 100 children he sees every week in his clinic, approximately half were potty before the age of three and are so-' dysfunctional voiders,' because of which urinary tract infections, bed weathering, and sudden occurrence of accidents (regression) have been caused. When a child holds poop chronically, a mass forms in the rectum that fills up the space that the bladder uses to retain urine, the nerves may be irritated by the mass and trigger involuntary contractions of the bladder.

Unwanted contractions, together with a lack of urinary capacity, frequently cause urination and accidents.

It's getting even stressful. This collection of poo in the rectum includes several bacteria. And that bacteria are very likely to glide over the bladder and trigger bladder infections in children, mainly if they are inclined to pee. You're not alone if you're cringing about all this pink and poop talk. Some parents think that potty education is healthy and does not bother to mention it to their doctors. Nonetheless, it must be addressed. The prevention of injuries, bed weeding, and bladder infections have been the main focus of recent studies, including this one released by the National Center for Biotechnology Knowledge.

How are these problems related to early training?

The reason small children who train potty as early as the age of 2 have more issues than children who wait for at least three years is that they are not mature enough to decide for themselves when they will pee and pee. You do not know yet how necessary it is to remove right when you feel the urge and eliminate it. According to Dr. Hodges, the bladder shrinks every year while retaining urine and is overactive.

What are you supposed to do?

Tell your child every two hours to use the toilet. Don't ask. Don't ask. We are probably too busy to have fun and keep it as long as possible. This is a dangerous habit, which strengthens the bladder to such an extent that the child is desensitized to sensations of fullness, and the bladder empties itself. Don't bow to the burden of peers. When a school or daycare provider advises you that your child needs potty education before going to school, find another provider.

Remind them to "let it out" before leaving the bathroom. You may be a lucky parent whose child just "gets it" off the fleece. Right, maybe your child is two years old. But remember that you are not alone, with parents still dealing with potty training. Finally, you're in the majority.

You don't trust a baby to brush its teeth every night, and you don't trust a baby to know how to extract them every time you use your shower. Recall early potty training can extend your duty to track your bathroom habits closely.

Additional potty training resources: risks of early potty training interaction of toilet age and incomplete voiding.

Potty training should be a tried-and-tested experience for both the child and the parents. Progress typically does not occur without accidents— and potentially tears or other setbacks — on the road. Understanding how to use the toilet does not suit any effort in one size. Whatever your potty training experience, it is essential to ensure that your child feels comfortable and that you express a positive attitude when learning this new skill.

While positivity is the answer, you need to know those "don't"— and avoid falling into them. Below are some of the most common well-meaning yet ultimately ineffective pitfalls for clearing your child while training potty.

Do not push the issue. Make sure that your child can use the pot before training begins. A child who can express their needs demonstrates interest in bathroom independence and is capable of meeting the physical needs such as shoes, knowing when "they need to go," and following a series of necessary steps is common signs of preparation. If you think that your child may not be ready, allow them a few more weeks or months before you try again.

If your child refuses to leave, it may create a negative atmosphere to force them to go and sit on the pot and eventually lead to more resistance. This can create detrimental associations with using the bathroom that can be difficult to eliminate and create your child to refrain from urination, which can be harmful.

Often seek to provide support and encouragement. If the process becomes a fight, even if your child seems "ready," otherwise, you could consider breaking. If you are both excited about this "big baby" move, you will get the best results (with potty training and relationship).

Try to treat this phase of learning just as you do with other milestones such as sit, walk, and speak. Honor, though almost all children arrive there, others need a little more time and maturity to master these skills.

You should not start training during a time of stress. Even good stress is weak stress when it comes to potty training. Marriages, new children, vacations, guests, and vacations will trouble your child–including the difficulties of coping with divorce, death, or moving to a new home.

If something new and significant is on the horizon of your life, rethink potty training right now. Wait before life settles, and the healthy activity flow begins again. It gives your child protection and allows them to position toilets alongside other regular routines quickly. Moreover, you will receive more focus and positive energy to help your child recover from the pains.

Don't set deadlines. Young children sometimes aren't working well within periods and don't have the same time definition as adults. Keep the potty training goals practical. Or, better yet, drive them out the window. Know that potty children train at different levels and ages. Some children learn before eighteen months but may take another year to a few years before they are ready. Before just before kindergarten, some don't master the skill. While some kids train the toilet quickly, it's a much longer process for others.

Programs that pledge that in three days, a day, or even 100 days, your child will receive potty training, do not take into consideration your child's individuality. And the child has a unique personality and development goals and brings various skills to the table, and there is no clear one-size-fit solution.

Programs operating on schedule frequently recommend corrective interventions, or are inflexible or train parents (as when your child watches any ghost or takes your child any 10 minutes to the bathroom), instead of the kid. This sets the deadline for a feeling of disappointment and lots of unhealthy tension for a lot of parents and children.

However, the many diverse social households, including working parents, households with loads of children, children with special needs, multiples, and parents with custody, can not be taken into account. Make sure that every approach you use is versatile and meets everyone's needs. Particularly, choose a potty training strategy that will encourage your child to feel comfortable, no matter whether it takes a few days or several months.

Don't view accidents as a big deal. One of the cornerstones of useful and productive potty training models is to remember: "It's a regular part of life." Make your child more confident: going to a bathroom — and the sometimes occurring accident — is inevitable and nothing to feel terrible about. Accidents happen, and as part of the planned process, we learn from them.

In reality, overemphasis on accidents can exacerbate misfortunes or feelings of shame, which lead to more accidents. If they arise, keep the tone calm and slow, or even arrogant. Recruit your child in the clean-up and proceed to the next opportunity to use the potty.

Don't wear clothing that is hard to deal with an instructor who is in charge of a group of potty trainees who can tell you how difficult buttons (snaps, zips, socks, overalls, several layers, and several other unmanageable clothes) can be controlled for little arms and hands.

Make it as convenient for your child as possible. Use the child's motor skills as a guide when choosing potty clothing. Simple pants, shorts, or skirts in the elastic waist are ideal for most people.

Shy away from overalls unless your child can remove and restore them. The same applies to suspension belt, belt, tights, single-piece shirts, and everything with plenty of zippers, snaps, buttons, or other fixtures, which might be a challenge to handle quickly and independently from your child. If you are at home, consider allowing your child to run in underwear or nude if you are confident. It is the ultimate potty training gear, after all. Most parents support this approach, as it works very well if our child wants to go to the bathroom (or just missed) straight away.

Since winter is the season of blankets, packages, and heavy coats in colder climates, most experts and parents believe that it might not be an ideal time for potty training. During the summer, children with bathing trunks or two-piece bathrobes have made it through potty training. Children in one-piece suits face a more significant challenge (mainly when they are wet). The choice of swimming outfits with a separate floor makes removing when needed easier.

External pressure can not be permitted to emerge from several outlets (in terms of how and when potted trains and how easily outcomes can be achieved): grandparents, other playgroup members, pre-school managers, teachers and partners. Bear in mind that while others may be full of childcare wisdom, sure advice may not resonate with you or work best for yourself and your child. Go with your intuition and focus on the information you have about the readiness of your child and the strategies that make you (and your child) the most convenient.

Whether intentioned or not, it is easy for our children to feel threatened, less threatened, or competing with other parents around the house. Recall that the vast majority of children learn these skills — they all learn at their own pace, at various times. Resist stressing about who learned potty first or best or most comfortable. Necessarily, it doesn't matter because you may only feel overwhelmed or simply evil.

Don't follow school schedule Schools blindly, which require your child to be potty and educated for a certain age, may simply meet licensing requirements, or escape discomfort. Licensing requirements allow any room with a child in slides to be equipped with a changing table and a sink and other supplies. When the classroom has hot water at a temperature different from that of the bath, the school will use a separate heater to operate new plumbings.

Schools may not have the trouble to outfit a room, or they may not want to spend money. Think this way, if the school already sets an arbitrary time limit for toiletries and does not take account of each child's individual needs, which other areas will this thought apply to? If this is your school's reality and you have choices, it may be worth wondering if this is the right school for you or your kids.

Don't wait for nighttime exercise. Right Usually, urinary control takes place before bowel movements are regulated, and the dry nights go well behind both. Betting (or enuresis) in children is common until they are four years of age or older.

About 20% of 5-year-olds and up to 10% of 7-year-olds are bed weathered, according to the American Academy of Pediatrics. Bladder control happens years later during the night for many children, and bed temperature doesn't necessarily mean a medical problem. Know that even healthy children often use pull-ups or wet beds in primary school, so don't hesitate to speak to the pediatrician if your child is worried. The vast majority of the body gains more urinary regulation naturally— it takes time.

The AAP lists two key factors: the bladder of your child may not be able to retain urine for the whole of the night, or it couldn't be noticed when he or she needs to go to the toilet and wake up. This is a four-step procedure for a child who is asleep. Some children are so lazy that they don't wake up until it is too late.

Confident that your boy will ultimately get there and not stressing it as an "issue" helps your kid know that what they are feeling is natural and nothing to be ashamed of so that it will help speed up the process.

Don't underestimate your child's fears or attachments. Children will develop fears and fears as much as the fears of adults during pottery training. Children can also be afraid of something you never thought about as an adult. The main thing is to respect your feelings and to care about them.

Children can not understand the workings of the toilet, and the noisy flushing sound may be disturbing in this small room. When a kid just has a fall off the toilet, and the water can be put on one square or even needs a potty training session. Some kids fail to see their dick vanish down the stream as though it were part of them as much as an arm or a leg.

Act with empathy for these fears. Discuss your anxiety without invalidating it or making your kid feel unimportant. Many kids may need help voicing their thoughts and coping with their emotions, so give them the right vocabulary.

The same applies to attachments that children will display during this period. Diapers may reflect a sense of safety or a "private" kindergarten. This is a time when parents are close to their children and take care of their needs, and allowing individual children to do so takes more time.

This does not mean you have to give up your exercise or let your child go back and forth between wearing slides and training whenever they want, but it does mean that they are ready. If your kid appears to want to cling to the diapers, it is high time to give them a story (regardless of whether they have used the potty or not) on your lap, a tickle, or some fun activity. This may not be your missing child's diaper, but its proximity to you. After all, it can be cold and lonely in the shower.

A Verywell Word Don't worry too much. You have heard or read that a million times now, but it's true: your child is doubtful to go to school in a windscreen.

Try to learn potty step by step and work with your kids. Find it yet another learning experience and another step in the life of this unique person's growth and freedom. Treat your child with the same compassion and motivation that you would want in the same situation, and don't forget to have fun.

TIPS FOR POTTY TRAINING: 6 ROUTINE PARENT TECHNIQUES

Potty training is difficult. Some teachers shared their advice to make potty training easier.

Children are having brand new characteristics as they start to fly to daycare. To learn more about day-care workers and their unusual abilities, I have asked several early childhood teachers around the country for tips for potty training. First, they acknowledged that having no parent of a child has its advantages. "We've got a different relationship with the baby. We will hold the thread, "says James Barker, site manager at the Kids & Company Front Street location in Toronto.

Daycare staff tend not only to be firmer than parents; they often have less concern and are never hurried into the bathroom. Vivian Turner, Executive Director of the Edmonton Garneau University Childcare Centre, says, "Parents need to relax. "A tiny adult is walking in a slip." Here are some more in-depth tips on professional potty training: a lot of daycare training convincing a kid to sit in the pot is no easy feat. Some are scared, some get mad, and some don't care. "I'm going to carry a child's friend who's educated in the bathroom, and let that child go first," Barker said. Then he recommends that the untrained boy try it. If the child refuses, Barker shrugs it–and offers it a couple of hours later again. And the next day, and the next day. "We don't force it if they hesitate," Barker says. "But, we inquire regularly." The potty process is broken up into phases at Moore Place Day Care in Georgetown, Ont. Next, a child is told to pull his or her pants down (and then up) in the bathroom. "They have to consider what goes first logically," says Carol Bee, Managing Director of Moore Place, adding that children who can do this themselves save staff time. Flushing toilet paper or pulling toilet paper allows children to feel in control of the bathroom environment. Most daycares do have a series of potty books to help children get acquainted with this concept.

Try this at home:

You don't have some small children to place peer pressure on, but you can use an older sister, relative, or friend to display the joy of using the bathroom. And try to hide your anger when you get a stubborn no to your bathroom offers. Yet continue to bid. Start to adjust your child's slide in the bathroom and suggest small activities, including pulling down your socks, taking down your toilet paper, and flushing. If he finally shoots him, show him you're happy and excited, even if he doesn't punch or fuck.

1. Will I go to plastic or porcelain?

The daycare way: the controversy between potty and toilet does not seem to be very common at daycares–they have what they have, and children have to adapt. "It's a little obstacle, but we're working around it," Barker said. If they all have toilets of full height, daycare staff will pull out stools to help children step up. Wonder why don't you see many preschool toilet inserts? They're difficult to keep clean, so most daycares avoid them.

Try it at home: Daycares can not meet the individual needs of each child, but you can have more flexibility at home and take advantage of it. Toilets are large and noisy, and some children are frightened; others know that potty is not what adults use and give them a snub. Therefore you have a potty and a seating area available (decorated with Dora or whatever appeals) and use the one your kid wants without making a pitch or attempting to speak to her as relaxed as possible.

2. Accidents occur while potty training takes place.

The way of daycare: "This is an accident; it's not premeditated," Turner says. When a child who is taught potty falls into his pants, daycare staff see this as a regular part of the training phase. They clean up quickly, put the child in fresh clothes, and just move on. At the same time, when there are incidents, workers will seek to assess if it is caused. "Sometimes the child doesn't feel well," Turner says. Or a significant change, such as a new baby, renovation, or holiday, may trigger a range of setbacks. "They'll be dry again if they're dry at one point," Turner says.

Try it at home: remember it's a temporary process, and your child will go back to the toilet. Seek not to get angry or blame her for retrogression. If you think the relapse is the product of something happening around her, speak to your child to see if you can help her cope.

3. What to treat honors and commendations.

The way of the daycare: "We have a sticker in the bathroom, so when they sit down and want to go, you can put a sticker on your own," said Anne McKiel, director of YMCA's Dartmouth Childcare in Dartmouth, NS. Some day cars make a lot of use when a child uses the toilet by loving him and sharing the news with his other friends.

Try this at home: Build a reward program that will empower and support your kids. Barker learned that parents give their children every time they go to a Hot Wheels car–it's a little. Instead, try stickers or checkmarks. But think about making your reaction a great motivator. "Mom says' Good work' with a huge smile and hug is also the best reward," says Turner.

4. Timing is everything.

Daycares have their approach to planning a ride to the bathroom. Daycare staff at Kids & Company execute a bathroom routine four times a day. At Moore Place, the staff takes children to the potty every half hour in training. Center McKiel leaves things very open. "We are watching the kids and having the plan for them," she says. The challenge, all three-day cars say, is for children to stick to them. "It is tough for children to abandon what they do," Barker says. Daycare workers also warn children that a break in the toilet is approaching, which reassures them that their toys will stay until they come back.

Trying it at home: Set your potty schedule at home according to your child's daycare schedule. When you're home full time, set your day and when you feel that your child will go more often. And just like daycare: let your child know in advance that it's almost potty time and then playtime goes on.

5. What should they wear?

Daycare: If possible, stop training slides. "A pull-up wall is the same as wallpaper, and children believe they can do the same thing," said Bee. Most daycare workers agree: go to underwear directly. Kids can still sense when they are soaked in underwear and, Turner notes, "most kids like underwear instead of pull-out painting." Barker wants, on the other hand, to wear a training slide on underwear for around two weeks of training.

Try this at home: while you may want to wear a diaper at night, underwear is the best way to learn seriously. Rush on Tigger or Cinderella undies— for some children, it is a real motivator. And you don't have to slip a training cloth over underwear for long drives or outings in your car. Your kid may always know, so you're not going to have to change his clothing.

6. Look out for number two.

Daycare: If children take time to research in the bathroom, daycare workers don't sweat. This also happens when a kid figures out how to urinate — perhaps a long time later. Bee knows of children who hide in the corner to fill their pains and anxiety to go to the toilet; they are also worried about getting in trouble or losing part of their bodies. Most daycare staff see this as a waiting game: they continue to offer the toilet, encourage children, and celebrate when it happens.

Practice it at school: Most children are keeping their bowels until, though, they get to school. If you know the usual routine of your kid, try to capture it with a toilet visit. Get her to read a book concurrently— it's confusing, and she could poop without knowing it. Even if it takes several months for a poo in the toilet to happen, don't sacrifice your coolness. Yet please make sure your child is congratulated when she goes.

Owed or not?

Between two and three and a half years, your child should be ready to begin the toilet workout. Here are several signs that he can take seriously:

• Remain dry for a long time.

• Showing interest in someone going to the bathroom.

• Ask for socks.

• Want protection when his diapers are packed.

But if your kid uses the potty during the day, it can take up to one year to dry during the night. Most children will wear undies around the clock in kindergarten. Both deciding factors are the duration and depth of your kid's night. It is the first approach to try: cut drinks after 6 pm.

THE TRUTH ABOUT EARLY POTTY TRAINING AND SHOULD YOU DO IT

Most children should be conditioned in the toilet by three or three and a half. If she succeeds in school, I'd speak to you about how you get her to go. Are all kids going at those times? Is there any kind of performance or keep dry? Then try replicating it at home. Setting a schedule can help some children (i.e., we get up at home and sit on the potty, then sit at the pot before dinners, snacks, and bedding) Try to maintain a positive experience and don't ask if it "needs to leave" just say "it's time to go potty." If she succeeds, reward her with love and small delicacies. Buy a few little toys one at a time from the shower curtain and tell her she can have them at bedtime while she's dry all day. After a few days of progress, make it two days for the toy and three days after.

One of the many positive things about a nice girl is that it's easier to prepare. Girls usually prepare for training earlier than boys and respond more quickly to instructions. Your work is now much more straightforward.

Once she's ready to be raised, your little girl will let you know. It will happen at the age of eighteen months. Often it can happen later, but that's no cause for concern. When the baby girl can stay dry for more extended periods, and be able to express movements, take them to begin a potty training for the baby girl.

A word of warning, it is imperative that you start when you trust the comprehension and motor skills of your child. Don't rush to train your child's toilet or backfire.

Training a girl in potty use is not very different from the training of a boy; flexibility and understanding are required in both cases. And you can gain a a lot of valuable tips from parents online forums who teach potty to their little girls successfully. Much of the time, you find that most tips speak of positive changes that can work well for the morale of the small child.

The cycle includes being alert to the need to go to the toilet for the infant. Take the girl to the bathroom, help her out, and sit down on the potty. A few things to remember: stop the child wearing extravagant clothes unless it's cold. Kids may not be able to maintain muscle balance until they get to the toilet after long pants and underwear are removed.

Small children's preparation is never an easy job to do. Most parents use diapers for most kids who undergo potty training during the night. It gives your child a bit of protection during the night and helps them to concentrate during the night on the most important thing.

To look for signals that prove your kid knows what he is doing, he will talk to you when they're wet or when he feels it's time to go to the loo. That's a sign they're ready.

As a mom, you need to know that girls 'potty training is a different activity than it is for men. In a family setting, the potty teacher is usually the woman nine out of ten, and little girls find it easier to learn from someone who they can imitate; the same is said for boys. If you have an older brother or your small boys 'dad in your family, ask him to go to the toilet with him so he can learn by modeling.

Most parents find it fun and enjoyable to use prizes and incentives during potty training to improve their child's behavior. Another perfect way to improve your little girl or boy's successful potty training is to use a set of photos.

You can pick up these in your nearest department store or a shop like Mothercare or even a bookstore. The books will be fun. These books or cards will demonstrate the entire cycle of using the potty and executing the operation. You should also let your child look at them when they are potty.

A few things to remember as potty girls are practicing-see that they are sitting erectly on the potty and not leaning over. Spraying is less a problem for girls than for boys. Hygiene, however, deserves special consideration. Girls are vulnerable to urinary tract infections. Little girls may not be able to self-cleanse, and the parent must ensure that after using the potty, it is clean. Get a potty with a seat too so that the child can learn to use it with the seat from the start.

After six months of intensive training, your little girl will have the potty ready; you'll need to be there with her before she can use the potty independently. In any case, when the young man is ready for pre-school, her diaper dependency will be surpassed.

Your 2-year-old isn't potty train yet.

The definition of potty training is to recognize the urge to go and the need to be clean... and then the potty. She needs not remain there long to excel.

Many kids don't need time to read the sports list. If they have to go, they're off. Check for the cognitive skills required to go to the potty and try again. Most parents have a couple of wrong beginnings before success.

I would advise you to quit a bit (as best you can!) at this stage. You don't want the potty training of your daughter to be turned into a fight for power. I will consider giving potty reminders. You want to follow the directions of your daughter and direct her. You want her to believe her entire idea was potty training. Yet support her and make her succeed. Have a potty she can reach everything on her own (she needs no help or a stool). Have a stack of clothing and a stack of clothes/training pants and let HER pick what she wants to wear. Continue with the conversations and excellent modeling (speak and let her see). Just don't push it into the shower, or put it on the toilet if it isn't her idea. Eventually, (actually, I hope sometime before college) she will try potty training on her own. She starts on the road when it's her idea and time, and the right day for her. As complicated as it is, the only thing you can do is let her lead.

How can I resist taking off my nearly 2-year-old daughter's slide at all times? I've taken her to her potty, but she sits down there and doesn't do anything, but she does take off her slide and (I know, gross) wants to play, dirty, or wet in it. Usually, she's not getting far before I catch her, but she's going to do this in her room.

Your baby is not potty train-ready, so don't make it easy for her to take off her clothes. One solution: tape loop. You won't be able to strip when you cover the diapers with duct tape. Or, you can make her wear overalls or remove other clothing similarly tricky. Bottom line: keep her from getting her bottoms off until she's ready for a toilet to run.

How do I get my two years of age to tell me she's going to have to go potty before she does it?

She may or may not be conscious at the age of 2 until she goes to the toilet. The first step to letting her know when to go or when she is gone is to get rid of the pull-ups and make her wear underwear. Pull-Ups remove the damp feeling that can allow you to know you ought to have gone to the toilet.

Scheduled potty times will also help to assess the use of the toilet. Start as soon as she wakes up in the morning and sits on the toilet every 2 hours a few minutes. Celebrate the successes and be able to wash a lot of wet clothing before she knows it.

My daughter is a heavy sleeper and does not usually wake up to use the toilet at night. Have you any ideas on how she should use the toilet at night?

If the bladder is full, the capacity of the brain to "wake up" is a developmental achievement at various ages. Some kids will figure it out during the day, but it's normal not to be dry at night until they reach seven years of age. You can't sadly "teach" her to wake up by wearing her panties and hope she's going to wake up because she'll feel wet. Each morning you just end up with a disappointed kid and a wet bed. If your daughter is old in school, start with reducing the intake of fluids or stopping fluids after dinner so that urine is minimized overnight. There are some behavioral training and bedwetting alarms for children around seven that can be successful, but they do not work for younger children.

My 34-month-old girl is popping off, and anytime after about 20 months, she feels like it. She never peed at the potty and now fails to come to tell me she has to go but then goes into her drawing. I've tried all the bonuses, but nothing works. Was anyone aware of how this stubbornness can be overcome?

A 34-month-old child is likely to be very reactive with emotions, so cajoling, complaining, and insisting on a specific action have reduced success levels.

You are right; I'm sure the problem is not that they don't grasp the concept of the grown-up toilet but that they are' stubborn.' Trying to be stubborn in the other direction won't help you— a boy will still win a power struggle. You can trust it! You can trust it!

Your best tactic is to get away from the war against the government. You have not tried to get your daughter to walk or talk or eat with a spoon or words. Those things were natural as their ability to understand expanded and their thoughts on how the adults were doing things contributed — of course — to their willingness to do the same. Kids can see that babies use a blanket, and adults use the toilet. Many young children want to use the toilet and use it successfully, especially if the parent encourages them a little with helpful ideas on how to do it.

When there is a power struggle, the inherent urge of the child to avoid being forced around is far greater than the need of the child to copy what the adults do. Then the child is dead and refuses the parent, even if it means continuing to kid. The fight can then become a trend that is difficult to change.

The only way to resolve the war of will is to fight for a while. Show your daughter as comfortable as she is and let the potty training issue run for many weeks. Then you should start giving her some kind suggestions for the use of the toilet after the war has subsided and she has forgotten it. I would approach her with respect and support like you would ask an older adult if she would be able to assist them with heavy packages or give them a seat in the metro.

Small kids want to do things the same way the people they love and admire are doing. This is the most potent motive for their growth. The reward is proud to be like the parents. Going for this inspiration is the best friend of the parent!

My child is 2 and 1/2 years old, and when she was two, she started pottery training. She's good with her potty chair at school. Often she wakes up if she's going outside the house anywhere. She is in daycare but wearing pull-ups because she won't say she has to go to a daycare class.

The daycare teacher sends her to the bath, and she still goes, but she only pulls up when the teacher does not take

her. She's not talking all that much yet, but she might say potty. How am I going to do?

What you describe is super-usual for potty kids. Children usually begin to blend potty rules with their relaxed and familiar home environment. These laws take a little longer to generalize to other areas such as school or the park. Savvy preschool teachers understand this and offer supplementary assistance and reminders at school. It usually is everything you need to know how to stay clean and dry at school. As her communication abilities improve, she can also express her needs better. Hang on!

My 3-year-old daughter has been practicing potty for almost a year. She has recently begun to keep up her need to pee (not to be distracted from whatever she does) so that she wets her underwear to wait. She eventually gets the desire to go again, but she's soaked her pants already. I tried to tell her to go the minute she feels the urge, but she refuses to do so. For example, there were also some injuries.

It's not uncommon for a child to start an accident after being trained because they're "too distracted." The other explanation may be that the optimistic enhancement of the performance of the toilet has also vanished. You will have to go back to the bathroom every two hours and avoid all the action before she gets back to the routine of doing it when she wants to go. Another way would be to celebrate "warm days" with every good day with a sticker chart and a seven days ' allowance for a couple of weeks. So spread the reward over a couple of cycles every 14 days and then monthly, and it will hopefully be back in the habit. If the events tend to be happening more frequently, a visit to the doctor's office might also be required if there is no urinary tract infection.

I guess my 18-month-old daughter is set for potty training. She still takes her paint when it's dirty; she knows what "potty" is and where the bathroom is.

She's been in the toilet a couple of times. What I'm not aware of is how much I will take her pot and how I can blend in or consider the demanding needs of a newborn. Any assistance or tips will be perfect!

I assume the word parent comes from the Latin word parents, which means "How many things will I do all at once?! "When it's time to teach a child potty, the parent must sure a child is ready and capable. Yet we forget that the parent must be ready and capable as well. Throughout parents ' lives, it often takes too long to make the effort and discipline necessary to teach a child. Even if a child is young (I would say less than three years), a parent can want to wait until the circumstances improve to the point that the parent has more time, resources, and the chance to do the job well.

When a child is willing, but the mother can not make a full effort, then she can still encourage the child to step in the right direction. For example, a parent may wish to give a child a chance to go potty, if the child wishes and encourage the initiative, but not push the child (or herself) to do so.

Alternatively, mom should only select a suitable time of the day for potty training (for instance, a time when the child still wants to bite pee alternatively) and concentrate on that time of the day only. If the child masters potty, the parent can then choose to do the same again.

My daughter was adequately potty trained at the age of 3. She had a stomach virus reversal. I allowed her to step back and think when she was ready, she would resume. She's four now, and she doesn't want to do it because "only big girls using the potty, and I don't have to go to school." I agree that I have two issues. Then I want to combat the potty war until I have school issues.

Help, please! She's pulling up in the least amount!

As a dad, I completely appreciate the disappointment that must be brought on. As a counselor, I am attempting to analyze the problem by disregarding anger and trying to answer those questions. Without learning more about the case, it's difficult to determine her remarks about the way' only broad girls use the potty.' She may have picked up her vocabulary and told you about big girls. So I'm sure that would be a reaction because it seems alarming. After all, indeed, you look at the potential consequences when it gets older.

Nevertheless, your daughter may not have been adequately prepared to be potty trained. Children who are really potty trained want the potty to be used. If she has repeated incidents and doesn't seem concerned, she may not have been ready at 3, and then the infection and the' step back' are snowballs. Without a medical condition (which a pediatrician can assess), she may need a little more time and a little less reaction from you. My sister's situation with their son was very similar, and they spent hours washing undies in the shower, and they felt all quite crappy. Progress was reached when my sister took a step back and reassessed her pain. We spoke about "he's not going in slippers down the aisle" and found that the less time we spent in the bathroom, the more he wanted to go, and the more he invested. As for education, I continue to speak to all children about their' jobs,' which are family members, have fun and go to education. Modeling what is anticipated (going, meeting people, and finally breaking away from your mother) will be your key to helping her succeed.

Using clothes is a luxury, not a privilege. That is until you prove you're ready to wear underwear, you can't wear underwear. Because only if you have an injury, can you prove it. If your daughter consciously has the need to go and then does it on your kitchen floor — she means that she doesn't have to be ready for this role instead of going to the bathroom. Go back a while to slides and try potty training again on the road for a weekend if she's ready, okay, then! Yet put her back in slides if she has accidents again. Many parents have many wrong beginnings before their child is ready. No concerns.

What can I do to support my 2-year-old son, who's potty ready, but fears it? I've got his potty chair, but he is always terrified of sitting on it without an underwear diaper. Why do I not scare my 2-year-old son from the potty chair?

It is growing insecurity— which can be reduced only by time, support, and space. Let your son discover the potty— both the large and the tiny ones— by himself and in his own time. He needs to "clone" how others use the potty, and his innate ability to use the potty starts in. I am having a lot of problems with Heather Wittenberg with my 3-and-a-half- year-old and the potty. A little before he was three years old, he began using the potty daily and, while he had no pants, he had a good handle when he needed to go. Within four months, he also started to experience injuries.

Sometimes he goes without injuries for a week or two, but instead, he gets injuries for three weeks every day. I don't understand why this happens. I don't understand. How is my son confused about going potty?

There are many explanations for delays in toilet training. Many children are so distracted doing what they do that they don't pay attention to the temptation to go–before it's too late. Some children do well at home but hate public powers, so they keep them at preschool or when they are out. Some children have strong concerns about the potty or had a poor experience with it, so they can't go if they need to. Without full information about what your child has gone through, it is difficult to explain why he has failed. But I think underwear is a luxury, and not a right— that means, if he has too many accidents, he is not adequately trained in a bathroom, so he must remain in a slide until he is ready.

What's my child's best way to train potty? I just found that the preschool my child does not take children on slides, and I have not started teaching her! Now start, but don't wait for miracles. Talk to pre-school staff if you can send your child to a disposable cabinet. Many schools are open to the idea as long as they know that you are teaching toilets. And your daughter may want to use the potty more as she looks at her classmates.

Potty training Your little princess in 5 simple steps

Potty training is not always an intimidating task. And if you have a baby girl to raise, it simplifies the cycle and lightens the burden. It may be easier to teach girls to use this pot because mothers usually educate children and girls quickly to share the gender with the teacher.

Once you have been persuaded your little girl is big enough to use your bathroom, here are five tips that can support your little princess in no time: Step # 1 Start Early Morning: Ideal early morning potty practice. Catch the kid early in the morning to get her to sit on the potty. The children would not be hesitant at the moment, so ensure you make good use of the opportunity. # 2 Loyalty: Once your little princess is right in her first phase, make sure you love her for doing an outstanding job. It will motivate her every day to use the potty.

Step 3 Do not say no to slides and sliders. When you are chucking clothes to train your boy, don't give up using underwear, or your little one will get used to them. Alternatively, wear tissue underwear to differentiate between the comfort of dryness and the discomfort of damp or soiled.

Step # 4 Using Potty Often, an essential move during potty training would be to use the potty regularly. And when you note that after a while your daughter hasn't soiled her pants, take her to the potty and sit until she stays. Sometimes in accidents, let her sit on the pot and pour the pot in the diaper in the pot to show her where the pot will go.

Step # 5 Using Slides at night Finally, after a full day of potty exercise, excellent post on the above steps, give yourself and your child a good night's sleep using sliders. You would only need them on the first days of potty training, as your little princess would soon be well educated not to need them.

HOW CAN I TRAIN MY TWINS SIMULTANEOUSLY?

With twins, of course, two babies would be in a family. It also means you are doubling your work. Feeding and taking care of the twins require a great deal of planning along with a positive attitude and outlook for your kids. The twins will also be raised day after day in the area of potty training as a "one-child family." To make this success and to contribute to its growth, follow these tips for potty twins:

1) Buy two potties. You will have two pans, each with its potty. The bowels and the 'toilet time' are uncertain for your twins to ensure that each one has a potty. Whenever two of them decide to go to the potty, bring them in their potty at the same time. The two pots should be put near each other to watch over your children. Unless the pots aren't similar to each other, it is difficult for you to test them. You have to go to another room or place where you can locate the other potty. That's going to be tiring. Buy two pots as soon as possible and position them next to each other.

2) Current potty. One way to introduce the twins to the potty is to put the potty. It can be portrayed in a specific way. You should let them see the pot and demonstrate or explain how to use it. It should be shown to your twin girls that sitting on the potty chair is the right thing to pee and pee. This would be better for your twin boys to have a role model to teach them how to use the potty. Let them know it's a two-way operation. In any case, you can also encourage them to watch a video or read a potty and potty exercise book. We can quickly mimic what they see. Especially for visual students, they can

understand what they learned and do what needs to be done for potty training.

3) Read and write for parents. Learn and learn more about the tips for potty twins. It helps you to know what else you need to learn and what your experience lacks. This will also provide you with an insight into how to make potty training more exciting and enjoyable for twins to stop them from getting overwhelmed. Also, ask other parents who have mastered potty training for their children for guidance or information. Take notes because it will help your research.

4) Additional purification. As you have twins, double cleaning is essential to sanitize your room. Clean the house every day and vacuum the pots. The bugs are kept away, so potty training is healthier.

Potty twins can be demanding. If all of your children are eager to use the bathroom, it is just as possible that someone will only struggle with their twins to get your attention. To remedy this, you need to increase your patience and teach them to do turns–not an easy task at this age. First, track your turn to sit on the toilet (that will make it more straightforward with a chart). Sister A says that she must go potty. Test the map; take her to the toilet. If it's her turn to sit there, put Sister A on the toilet. When Sister B thinks she has to go too, tell,' It is Sister A's turning on the toilet. If you must go, you could use the potty chair, and when she's finished, you then turn on the toilet. "If Sister B's going into the temper tantrum, know it, but don't hide within. You might say something like, "I know you're crazy, and you're looking to sit down on the toilet right now, but it's your sister's turn. You can go in just two minutes." It's more than two minutes to... As the emotions of your children will be durable as they try to be on the first toilet, you will need to be firm and kind while you control the situation. You know or get off of the pot. Two will be happy when she leaves, and the other will be irritated as she is waiting. If your twins are against the potty chair, get creative and make it more attractive — try to dress up like a throne, say. No matter whether the toilet or pot is or twins, make sure you give equal credit (and prizes, if you use them). Remember, potty training is just one of the "turn-taking" tasks for your twins. Regardless of whether you turn on your computer, play the piano or later drive the car, you can't have two of them. In addition to the benefits of your girls having to use the bathroom, they also have the added advantage to share. —Team of parents

How to do a practical 3-day potty training is an integral part of becoming a mom. While this can be a daunting thing to do, potty training isn't as hard as other parents would think. It can be completed only in 3 days! Have your eyebrows lifted this statement? Do you doubt the idea of a 3-day potty training and think it's a bluff?

The goal of this is to show that parents like you can indeed manage 3-day potty training.

Early planning is also essential for the big day. Of starters, you can buy the potty and a few training pants and undies two weeks before the actual training begins. It also helps if you show and encourage your child to play with the app.

The idea is to make your little one more confident with the potty. Your pre- potty training ends the night before the first session. Remember that night; your child will be a big day tomorrow as he/she will be a big kid/girl. In the entire training cycle, there should be no distractions. Make sure your timetable is transparent so that you can completely commit to your baby's preparation for those three days.

Place the potty in an accessible area and ensure all other resources are ready on the training day itself.

Training

It takes a lot of effort, discipline, and dedication to making your child successfully learn. Yeah, it can be challenging, but that doesn't mean it's impossible. These are the ways to make it useful: greet your child's day with a smile and tell him cheerfully that he/she will pink on the potty starting today. Place the fresh undies on it. Shortly afterward, urge him to drink a big glass of milk or water to avoid peeing. Set a timeout and try to place your child every 15 minutes on the potty.

You should also expect injuries, apart from being concentrated. Patiently remind your child to pee or poop on the potty with should incident. Don't make your kid overwhelming. Praise him for all the successes.

Also, specific therapies like stickers or candy may yield more positive effects. Let your child know with every accomplishment that he/she does something beautiful and that you are happy about it. The preparation will take place all day long. At night, sleep pants are recommended.

Only try to do what you did on the first day. Based on your child's reaction to the instruction, you may adjust the time interval. For example, every 30 minutes, you can place your child on the potty instead of 15.

The last day of training is very significant as it determines the quality of your child's training. You should remove the use of a timer this day. Only ask your child if he/she has to pink. If appropriate, place your little one on the potty.

The Potty Training business demands patience and love.

6 Potty Training Tricks Fathers, who made the process simpler, can be very difficult. Here's how to make things a little more bearable, according to six days.

It is not shocking that potty training is one of the most challenging aspects of raising a child. It's overwhelming. It's annoying (the accumulation of one warrant). The good news is that when a child is ready to start potty training, parents can use several tricks to help them out. Many of these are not new, and it is not essential to reinvent a wheel that is thousands of years old, but it is worth listening to the tips of parents with recent achievements. It's comforting if nothing else.

1. At least three dads listed their experience with the Daniel Tiger Potty training episode. Watch Daniel Tiger Potty training episode. Titled "Daniel Goes Potty," it advises children to stop and go immediately. "We used this to teach my son potty, and it helped him a lot," Brian, a Rockland County, New York two-father, said. "It was instructive, indeed, but most beneficial was that it came from a character in whom he knew and connected.

2. Tot-on - the-pot as an innovative "play-based" potty training program features a soft doll and personal mini toilets, a detailed parenting guide, 20 laminated business cards, and a Tot on the pot board. Tot-on-the-pot is an innovative potty training program. The game was a perfect "Partner-in-Poop" for his daughter, Fatherly publisher Dave Baldwin said. It not only provides a kid with a potty break, but it also helps children conquer the toilet with game-based rewards. Other potty training games help with role-playing, too.

3. As potty boys learn, some dads vowed by turning potty training into target practice. Giving their son something to aim for–and having a game–helped him conquer the dresser. You can buy or build your targets online. "I draw boats and ducks on tissue paper, and the goal is to sink the target," one father said. This is a smart tactic, in any case, for people not only focused on time but also precision and freedom.

4. This board, where Elmo teaches little children about the art of making potty, is written not only in plain, straightforward, simple language, but also contains more than 30 interactive

articles that you can pull or push on each page. Many fathers reported how helpful the book was in introducing the idea of potty training and in encouraging and reassuring them.

5. "We traveled quite a bit when our first daughter trained potty; given how important consistency is, this was the greatest help," says Louisville's two father Kevin.

6. Make a choice and stick "Don't move between underwear and paints with it. We switched to underwear all day (including snack time), then to underwear at night (we call them underwear at night). The gap is enormous, and we do not use the toilet at any time, day or night, "one father said. If you start your potty workout, it may be tenting to have a transition period from slides to undergarments depending on the time of day. Yet it can confuse a child, and the decision to wear underwear all day, even during nap time, helped his child with the plan.

HOW TO POTTY TRAIN TODDLER

And for parents of stubborn children, this fear is even greater.

You know who you are. You know who you are. The day is one argument after another, and you are drained by night.

Which happens to this equation when you add potty training? It may be a tragedy... but if you follow our measures and take your time, you will be safe before you know it!

The worst thing you can do to continue with a stubborn child on this path is to start the process too early. They will not cooperate if they are not ready to begin.

Time. The power dynamic will be at work right from the start, and even though you pause and take a break for one month, you will remember who won the game. Trust me. Most children can start potty training between the age of 2 and slightly after their third birthday, with boys in this time zone coming later. Around 50% of boys are trained for three years, while 66% of girls are trained for three years. Kids with special needs are more likely to train later.

Do not try to rush through the process when your child is too young. The American Association of Pediatrics states that children who start potty training at 18 months of age are still not fully trained up to four years of age. Until well into their fourth year, several children can not tolerate bowel movements in the toilet.

When do I know my child's potty train ready?

Your child will show you the signs of their readiness. There is anything to look for: if the diaper is dirty, your child will tell you.

Your child is going to tell you right before or when he's leaving. During the day, their diaper stays dry for about two hours at a time.

Bowel movements occur frequently.

Your child usually stays dry throughout the night.

Your child can show toilet interest and underpants interest.

Because they are uncomfortable, your child can take wet diapers off themselves.

Before peeing or pooping, you may notice your child facing.

You will also see that your child is confident, wants to do something for himself or herself, and may enjoy some time alone.

If your kid is reluctant or scared of the toilet, whether he has an intestine or urine right after you have them sitting on his author, or wet their paint in less than two hours, he is not ready for the potty train.

How long is it going to take?

That depends entirely on your kids. For most babies, you can expect it to be a good two or three months before they are fully educated. This could take a lot, much longer for others, particularly children with special needs. Take a deep breath, put on your patient hat, and brace yourself for many injuries.

THE EQUIPMENT YOU SHOULD USE FOR SUCCESSFUL POTTY TRAINING.

The children of Stubborn will sense something going on before you tell them and will watch over them. Instead of attempting to start potty training like a sneak, involve them in the planning. Involved children are more likely to comply and less likely to see the entire thing as a problem for you.

Here are some fun ideas to get your kids on your potty training team: let your kid help you "practice" a pot or stuffed animal. You might also want to buy a drink and a wet doll with a tiny toilet so that your kid can experience drinking and then urinating.

Go out and have fun buying trendy clothing.

While in painting, have your child start to help with painting to make them more conscious of the process. Get a dry diaper for you, decide when to change your socks, pull socks up and down, and even scrub. Think about what you do and continue to talk about how long you're going to use the bowl.

Read fun toilet training picture books

Should not adjust them at once while your child is still in a diaper to begin to equate a sensation of discomfort with pains. It will also help them get involved because they may start asking you to change their wallpaper.

Let them see you in the bathroom, so they know that the toilet is used by adults and older siblings. Discuss how cool it is not to wear slides. Tell them they're going to have to use the toilet too soon.

Once you are ready to get going, load out your basket with slides worth two or three days and say, "These are the last slides. You will have to use the potty when these clothes are gone. That means your child will have a head up and an authentic sign of a potty training day ahead.

Here is the list of equipment required for potty training

Potty or training seat: It is essential to have a good potty seat. You want to make your child happy and feel safe in the potty. We like the potty seat Baby Björn that goes straight into the toilet, but some kids like to start on the ground. In that case, the potty chair of Baby Björn is a good alternative.

Step Stool: You would certainly want a step stool if you intend to make your child sit down on the toilet with a potted seat so that they feel comfortable and secure. Sitting high on your legs can feel scary and painful. A simple step hob will make a difference to your child and encourage them to feel comfortable in the bathroom.

Potty picture books: Put some potty books on your bookshelf and include instruction in your time of reading, too.

Underpants: have fun picking out the cartoon and bright underpants. Make a unique journey out of it!

Pants: These pants are more absorbent than standard underwear and can absorb minor leaks. These can be easily combined with vinyl pants between clothing and underwear.

Elmo's Potty TimePotty training cartoon videos: Many training videos are available that help boosts potty training through cartoons. We love Elmo's Time, Potty.

Beverage and wet doll: remember how fun you had these lifelike dolls? And they're also a great learning tool!

Sweatpants and other clothing that is simple to remove: You probably already have a beautiful set of clothes to fit your boy, but if not, now's the time to collect them. For example, some parents opt for potty training without shoes!

THE STEP-BY-STEP GUIDE TO POTTY TRAINING

Ok, maybe there's a potty training day! Ideally, your baby is still on board! Now is the time to take it easy, don't force it too hard, and get the bleach wipes out because you will need them.

Follow these easy tips, and you can easily remove diapers off your shopping list: pick a week that you can spend full time on potty training, such as spring breaks or winter holiday. Don't start training during a period of stress, especially at the birth of a sibling when children naturally return a little changed anyway. If you can eat it, try potty training during the summer, when your child can travel with little to no clothes more chill and relaxed.

If the time has come to sit on the potty, don't ask your child if he wants to go potty. Just carry him to the potty and sit on it.

Stay on the potty for 5 minutes or an acceptable period.

Set a timer for 30 minutes after sitting on the potty if he didn't potty, 1 hour if he did. Sit on the toilet when the timer leaves (so the timer is the one that says that you don't have time to sit on the potty).

Drink plenty of liquids.

Wear underwear and quick to put on and off clothing. Many potty parents only train their children with no pants to concentrate on the potty and not the clothing. If your child is entirely naked (at least on the bottom) for potty training, accidents would be even more noticeable to them. Summer is a great time to practice potty due to hot weather.

Here's a Fun Tip:

Put a few drops of food coloring in the pot and tell your child that the water will change into another color when she pees. And put the cheerios in the pot to see if your son can shoot and sink them.

Don't get worried about injuries (because some do happen). Only clean up and keep the day. You don't want your child to fear failure.

Praise is beneficial, but don't overdo it, because it may potentially add to the situation. You don't want your kid to feel like they have dropped you in an accident.

Aid the potty calm. One right way to do this is to make a calming potty poem. We sing: "Pee pee, pee-pee, it was time to get a pee-pee," lovely and soft and with a touch of "A ticket a casket." A big glass jar of M&M fits well as it's fun, and you can see the treat on the shelf waiting for you. A diagram with squares and adhesives is also fine. Don't forget too much support and hugs! That means that everything you give to be rewarded in the bathroom has to remain in the bathroom — no M&M all day long! Give a reward for sitting on the plate, even if you don't click, but if you pink, you offer a greater reward. Wean away the bonuses after a few weeks of functional pots. Start by missing the treat before your child reminds you–they will inevitably forget about that too.

Keep wearing pain for a while or on long trips. Don't think about the dry night when showing the potty to be used throughout the day.

Remember: relax and fast. Even if they're too stubborn, your child should know how to use the toilet. It will take some time, and you definitely won't pressure them or press them, but it will happen if they are ready for growth.

POTTY TRAINING CHALLENGES AND REMEDIES: AN EVIDENCE-BASED GUIDE

Typical potty training issues include fear and anxiety reaction to the inability of the potty to using toilet facilities outside the home and incidents. The challenges and remedies are not based on facts.

How can we do with these issues?

When we prepare ahead, several of them can be stopped in the first place. I give tips to avoid trouble at the end of this post.

But first, let's remember what you might do if you hit a stumbling block already.

Here is a guide to dealing with raising potty training issues based on facts.

1. Solving potty training issues induced by anxiety. It might seem that children are lazy or irrational if they declined to comply. Yet many children have reasonable reservations about toilet training. It's just the uncertainty of something different sometimes. The potty chair is unknown; that's the routine.

Children also have different toilet concerns. You may be afraid of the noises made by toilets or the mysterious disappearance of flushed objects. You may be scared to fall into the toilet or worry about the possibility that there is something inside— a bug or beast.

And many children have suffered constipation, urinary tract infections, or other medical conditions that have caused the toilet to be associated with discomfort.

Whichever trigger a child is trepidation, it is not beneficial to be coerced or pressured into toilet training. No one likes to be pushed and frogged by a mysterious operation!

Young kids will know what to do. You have to know that nothing can be afraid.

Therefore, if your child shows signs of anxiety about toilet training, this anxiety is reduced first.

Be sure your child does not suffer from constipation, tufted stools, and other potentially painful conditions until you try something else.

And even if you see no signs of a medical problem, the diet and fluid intake of your child is helpful. Make sure your child eats ample water and a high fiber diet.

And take the time to help your child learn: Tell your child what to expect and encourage your child to study and make questions.

Let your child get accustomed to the potty chair by leaving it where your child plays. Discard future concerns by describing how things work. Show, for instance, how your kid works and reassure him or her that there is nothing to fear.

When your child gets more comfortable, continue to incorporate "potty sitting" activities, where your child can sit on the pot for a short time.

Your child will remain fully clothed for the first few practices sits and sit for 30 seconds or so. Praise your child for working together.

As your child accepts the process more, you can practice your child bare-bottomed, and gradually extend the sessions.

Once you have overcome the fears of your child, your child will be ready for re-education

2. What to do when children fail to sit flat out; often, children do not sit on a potty chair or toilet. Too what?

Next, maintain the security and control of your child while he/she sits. When the feet of children are left sluggish, children are not merely less comfortable. They also have more significant trouble regulating their void muscles.

That is why experts say that toilet training is best achieved with a child's potty. Place a child's training seat on top of your toilet and put a small stool below your child's feet.

Secondly, consider the psychological preparation of your infant. Will your child need to know even more before moving ahead?

Pediatricians, like those of the CPS, say that rejection is an indication that the child is not prepared for training. You suggest that you refrain for a month or two from potty training and start again.

This suggestion is not unfounded. Trying to push a reluctant child through toilet training is a bad idea. Children can respond by attempting to retain urine or stool and increasing the risk of infection or constipation of the urinary tract. Another way to raise the anxiety and fears of your child is by manipulation–creating more potty training issues.

But you don't just have to wait. Use your time then to familiarize your child with the steps that people take to use the bathroom.

Fix the child's worries or doubts. Read picture books on the method, examples, and a positive attitude model.

Then, as the resistance of your child fades, you may implement the above-stated sits.

Don't let children sit alone, bored, without anything to do. Grant them friendship and diversion.

Read these evidence-based tips for more information on preparing your child for toilet training.

3. Treating children who would not poop The child is likely to urinate in a bowl or toilet but opposes bowel movement. What's going on? What's going on?

This is called "toilet rejection," and evidence suggests that it is related to constipation and painful bowel movements.

For example, one in four children had stool toilet refusals in a study that tracked 380 American boys, and in many cases, the problem was followed by constipation.

Furthermore, children with frequent hard bowel movements have been more than twice as likely to suffer from a refusal of a stool toilet.

When you struggle with stool rejection, it makes sense to pay careful attention to the diet and fluid intake of your child and to address the issue with your doctor.

If you can make bowel movement easier for your child, potty training issues for your child could be resolved early.

There is also evidence that a streamlined and encouraging way can help. Half parents were randomly allocated to take this approach in the sample of more than 400 young children– babies for defecating and the use of derogatory words for feces.

The method did not eliminate the rejection of the stool toilet but reduced the time required for children to develop out of it. It, therefore, seems essential to track how you interact with your child and to avoid communicating that defecation is shameful or disgraceful.

4. Resistance to toilets while your child is away from home Even adults will be unable to use a public bathroom, so it should not be challenging to feel empathetic. The most comfortable alternative is to use a portable toilet for children–the kind that can be placed over a regular toilet. Practice at home, and take it with you on your trip.

5. Daytime accidents understanding and bed wetting It is essential to be practical. Accidents during toilet training are prevalent! In reality, you should expect the occasional misfortune even after you have finished toilet training. The researchers described potting training in a study that tracks American children when parents registered "less than four urine accidents a week and two or fewer fecal soiling episodes a month." That's progress, but it's not right.

And the younger the child is, the better injuries can be prevented.

In a study that followed the development of about 60 Swedish children, researchers found that only 31% of 2-year-olds had an intense sensation of the bladder. In contrast, 79% of the 3-year-olds reported a bladder sensation. These researchers have found clues to the significance of bladder capacity.

Kids with higher bladder capacity at an early age tended to get dry day after day.

The accident rate of your child will depend both on his or her age and individual developmental factors. To prevent injuries, track the fluid intake of your child, and add some appropriate potted sits to your child's schedule.

How about the night?

The bladder requires a hormonal signal to generate less urine to remain dry at night. Sleepers will always feel comfortable with the bladder and only wake up when their bladders are fully felt.

On all these fronts, young children can face unique challenges: during early childhood, these abilities begin to grow. As a result, many kids don't hit the mark of nighttime dryness until they are 4 or 5 years old.

In the Swedish study, just referred to, for example, only half of the children were nocturnally dry by the age of 4.

So bed weathering is not as much a potty training problem for young children as it is a developmental process. Reducing fluids before bedtime will help, but nighttime incidents will not be prevented— unless your child has a mature bladder function.

Doctors are more likely to interpret this as evidence of concern when your child still wets the bed at the age of 5. Be proactive:

Ten tips to avoid potential potty training issues

Here's some more guidance on how to avoid possible mishaps and safety problems.

1. Prepare your child actively for potty education. As described in the introduction, by planning, you can prevent some potty training problems.

2. Stop confrontations explicitly. Do not force your child to sit or hold back your child when it wanted to get up yesterday, but suddenly resist your potty request. Your child cooperated yesterday. What should you do?

   Experts say that it's easier to get back and try later on. Coercion can lead to all kinds of problems, such as constipation, urinary tract, and phobia.

3. Don't encourage children to feel sad or bored. Seek to make your time on the pot by talking to your kids, reading stories, or playing games and toys.

4. Don't blame your child for injuries or scold them.

When children are disciplined or scolded, they may start refusing their urine

or stool, which puts them at higher risk for infections of the urinary system, constipation, and resistance to toilet stools.

5. Remove potty splash safety benches.

If they step on or off the potty, kids will catch their genitals. When you teach your son to pee, show him how to hold his penis down so that urine exits the potty. Let your son pee in a bucket if he likes to stand.

6. Take action for constipation prevention.

This has already been stated, but we must repeat: constipation increases the risk of the child having difficulties with potty training. Make sure your baby gets plenty of fluids (at least 4 cups a day) and takes plenty of fiber. Consult your doctor if your child has a chronic constipation problem.

7. Beware of the soapy water and bubble bath.

The soap can cause urethra inflammation, which leads to urination to pain. Girls are more likely than boys to develop this problem.

8. Do not allow your child to strain can lead to bladder and sphincter disorders. If your child can not urinate without pain, tell your doctor.

9. Try arranging a couple of potty routine day visits. Some doctors suggest that all potty sessions be initiated by children (not supported by parents). This approach is, therefore, a matter of personal choice. Another method involves daily potty breaks, such as after waking, after dinner, and before bedtime. If potty sessions are dealt with as part of the everyday routine, children learn to anticipate them without having to be trapped. Scheduled potty breaks can also be

useful for wellbeing, including avoiding infections of the urinary tract.

10.   Most children do not master wiping skills until 45 months of age. Helping your child clean For girls, good wiping is especially necessary. Since the women's urethra is shorter than the male urethra, the invasion of the female urinary tract by bacteria and infection is simpler. Teach girls to clean back and forth.